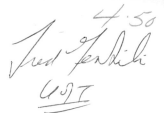

LECTURE NOTES ON OPHTHALMOLOGY

To
E. F. K.

LECTURE NOTES ON
OPHTHALMOLOGY

PATRICK D. TREVOR-ROPER
M.A., M.D., B.Chir. (Cantab)., F.R.C.S., D.O.M.S. (Eng.)

Consultant Ophthalmic Surgeon
Westminster Hospital and Moorfields Eye Hospital

FOURTH EDITION

BLACKWELL SCIENTIFIC PUBLICATIONS
OXFORD AND EDINBURGH

ISBN 0 632 08450 2

First published 1960
Reprinted 1961, 1963
Second Edition 1965
Third Edition 1968
Fourth Edition 1971

Distributed in the U.S.A. by
F. A. Davis Company, 1915 Arch Street,
Philadelphia, Pennsylvania

Printed in Great Britain by
Alden & Mowbray Ltd
at the Alden Press, Oxford
and bound by
The Kemp Hall Bindery

CONTENTS

PREFACE TO FOURTH EDITION

In many ways the practice of Ophthalmology has changed, even in the three years since our last edition, hence this further re-appraisal. But the overall pattern remains fairly constant, and this little book struggles to remain as slim as ever.

Patrick Trevor-Roper

3 Park Square West,
London NW1

PREFACE TO FIRST EDITION

THIS little guide does not presume to tell the medical student all that he need know about ophthalmology, for there are many larger books that do. But the medical curriculum becomes yearly more congested, while ophthalmology, still the 'Cinderella' of medicine, is generally left until the last, and only too readily goes by default. So it is to these harassed final-year students that the book is principally offered, in the sincere hope that they will find it useful; for nearly all eye diseases are recognized quite simply by their appearance, and a guide to ophthalmology need be little more than a gallery of pictures, linked by lecture-notes.

My second excuse for publishing these lecture-notes is a desire I have always had to escape from the traditional text-book presentation of ophthalmology as a string of small isolated diseases, with long unfamiliar names, and a host of eponyms. To the nineteenth-century empiricist, it seemed proper to classify a long succession of ocular structures, all of which emerged as isolated brackets for yet another sub-catalogue of small and equally isolated diseases. Surely it is time now to try and harness these miscellaneous ailments not in terms of their diverse morphology, but in simpler clinical patterns; not as the microscopist lists them, but in the different ways that eye diseases present. For this, after all, is how the student will soon be meeting them.

I am well aware of the many inadequacies and omissions in this form of presentation, but if the belaboured student finds these lecture notes at least more readable, and therefore more memorable, than the prolix and time-honoured pattern perhaps I will be justified.

ACKNOWLEDGEMENTS

My first thanks are due to my colleague, and formerly my teacher at Westminster Medical School, Mr. E. F. King, who kindly checked this book in proof, to Mr. T. Casey, who conbuted so many helpful suggestions for the first edition, and to Mr. Barrie Jay and Mr. Andrew Elkington for this fourth edition.

For the illustrations, I am particularly indebted to Dr. P. Hansell's Department of Medical Illustrations at the Institute of Ophthalmology, where most of the original drawings and photographs were prepared; and since the majority of these have already appeared in my textbook, *Ophthalmology*, I must acknowledge the help of Mr. Douglas Luke, of Lloyd-Luke, Ltd., its publisher, who readily made these blocks available. For the loan of other blocks I am indebted to H. K. Lewis & Co., Ltd. (Wolff's *Anatomy of the Eye*, Figs. 8 and 26), Ballière, Tindall & Co., Ltd. (May and Worth's *Diseases of the Eye*, by T. K. Lyle and A. G. Cross, Fig. 77; and Worth and Chavasse's *Squint*, by T. K. Lyle, Fig. 24); Longmans, Green & Co., Ltd. (Gray's *Anatomy*, Fig. 18); H. Kimpton (*Textbook of Ophthalmology*, by Sir S. Duke-Elder, Fig. 27); J. Wright & Sons, Ltd. (*Eye Surgery*, by H. Stallard, Fig. 30), Harvey & Blythe, Ltd. (*Brit. J. Clin. Pract. 10*, Figs. 3 and 11); Cassell & Co., Ltd. (Wolff's *Diseases of the Eye*, by R. Smith, Fig. 3).

My especial desire was that this book, in spite of its heavy load of illustrations, should be inexpensive, and well within the budget of those students for whom it was primarily written. This would have remained a pipe-dream had not the cost of the blocks been largely borne by certain pharmaceutical firms; and the generosity of Abbott Laboratories, Ltd., British Schering, Ltd., Ciba, Ltd., Merck, Sharp & Dohme, Ltd., Roche Products, Ltd., The Squibb Institute for Medical Research, and Upjohn of England, Ltd., will indeed be widely appreciated.

LECTURE NOTES ON OPHTHALMOLOGY

CHAPTER I

INTRODUCTION

To the ancients the eye was the gateway for the soul, and to the physician of to-day that modest organ indeed serves as a window through which the evidence can be seen of half the maladies to which man is heir. But the diseases specific to the eye itself are no less important, for the eye is exposed and vulnerable, and because man is primarily a visually-motivated machine, with an especial dread of anything that might lead to blindness.

The investigation of eye diseases is happily quite a simple affair. In the main there are only two presenting symptoms—loss of sight and pain; and since the affected tissues are so readily inspected, the front by a magnifying lens, and the back by the ophthalmoscope, the patient's subjective interpretation of his symptoms is of minor importance, and the diagnosis thus based on the objective findings of the surgeon can be comfortably exact and secure.

Eye diseases are readily grouped into two very different categories, separated by the tough outer wall of the eyeball.

The *external* diseases—such as those of lids and conjunctiva—behave like the many familiar diseases of skin and mucosa elsewhere in the body; they invite direct inspection, and are easily approached for a culture or biopsy; and they are equally amenable to topical treatment, since the drugs can be placed directly onto the affected cells, with rarely any danger of systemic poisoning, with maximal economy and with maximal ease; while minor operations again have easy access, rarely become infected, heal readily, and the results are most rewarding.

It is a very different matter when we deal with the *internal* eye diseases—those which affect the structures within that fibrous envelope. They can less easily be inspected, perhaps only darkly through a semi-opaque cornea or lens. They can be reached only with difficulty and danger for biopsy or culture, and even then the histological changes are often inconclusive, and the cultures negative; with the result that the aetiology of most internal eye diseases remains quite obscure. And finally, they are inaccessible for treatment, since—even if an effective agent were known—the corneo-sclera forms an impenetrable barrier to nearly all topical applications that are foreign to the body.

————

Before considering the specific diseases of the eye, a few words are needed about the eye itself, and the form and function of its several parts.

The **Eyeball**, a sphere nearly an inch in diameter, lies suspended within the orbital fat; it is protected by the four converging bony orbital walls, but unprotected anteriorly where the convex corneal window lies. The latter is screened by the upper and, to a small extent, the lower eyelids (Fig. 1); while a vestigial third eyelid lies immobile in the inner angle as a conjunctival fold (the 'plica semilunaris'), containing a fatty nodule known as the caruncle (well displayed in Fig. 17).

The **Cornea** differs from the **sclera** (which envelops the rest of the eyeball) primarily in being transparent and in being more convex (it is the cornea, rather than the lens, which is the major focusser of the retinal image). Its principal pathology lies in its liability to ulcerate, since it is exposed to all manner of traumata and of exogenous pathogens; and even if such ulcers rarely penetrate the whole corneal thickness, they leave opaque scars which, if centrally placed, may seriously impair the sight.

The cornea consists of a thin epithelium (five cell layers, corresponding to the three inner cell strata of the epidermis), a thick 'substantia propria' of laminated fibre-bundles (which

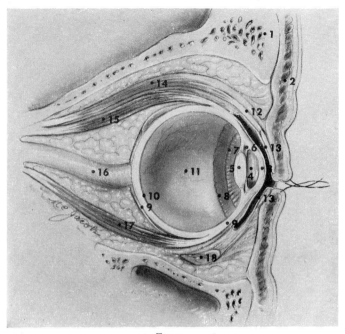

FIG. 1.

Vertical Section of Eyeball within the orbit. (From *Medical Radiography and Photography*, Courtesy of Camille Hill Killan.)

1. Frontal Bone (orbital rim).
2. Orbicularis Oculi Muscle.
3. Cornea.
4. Anterior Chamber.
5. Lens.
6. Iris Root.
7. Ciliary body.
8. Ora Serrata (anterior edge of retina)
9. Sclera.
10. Choroid and Retina.
11. Vitreous space.
12. Muller's muscle (involuntary; connecting L.P.S. and upper tarsal plate).
13. Tarsal Conjunctiva.
14. Levator Palpebrae Superioris Muscle.
15. Superior Rectus Muscle.
16. Optic Nerve.
17. Inferior Rectus Muscle.
18. Inferior Oblique Muscle.

continue into the sclera with little histological change, save for the presence of the episcleral blood vessels), and a single layer of endothelial cells in contact with the aqueous humour (Fig. 2).

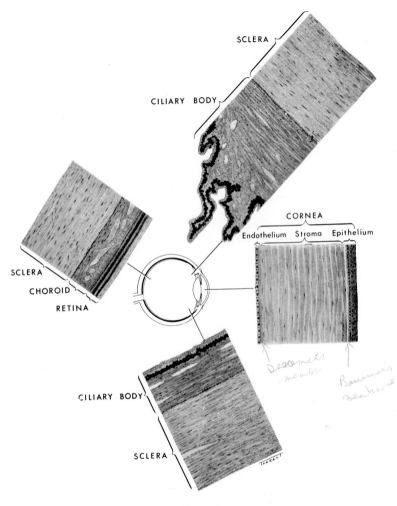

SCLERA

CILIARY BODY

CORNEA

Endothelium   Stroma   Epithelium

SCLERA

CHOROID

RETINA

CILIARY BODY

SCLERA

TARRANT

Desemets membr.

Bowmen's membrand

FIG. 2.

Histology of the coats of the eyeball.

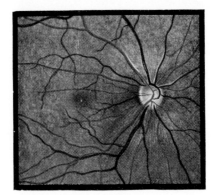

FIG. 3 (*see page* 5).
The Negroid Fundus. (Perkins and Hansell, *Diseases of the Eye.*)

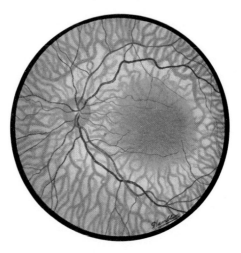

FIG. 4 (*see page* 5).
The Albinoid Fundus. (Hamblin.)

Lining the inner surface of the sclera is a mesodermal sheet known as the **'Uveal tract'**, loaded with blood-vessels and containing at its anterior end the unstriated intra-ocular muscles. Posteriorly this thin sheet is known as the **choroid,** and between its lattice of vessels lies a variable amount of pigment, so that on ophthalmoscopy of dark-skinned races the fundus appears chocolate in colour (Fig. 3); while in albinos the absence of pigment both exposes the wide interlacing choroidal vessels, and in the polygonal spaces between them reveals the white sclera (Fig. 4).

The choroid reaches forward to within 6 mm. of the corneo-scleral junction, and there the uveal tract becomes swollen by the fibres of the ciliary muscle, so that this intermediate zone is known as the **ciliary body** (Fig. 2). From ridges on the inner surface of the ciliary body, the fine fibres of the suspensory ligament of the lens pass centripetally to the latter's rim.

From the anterior margin of the ciliary body, the uveal tract is continued as the **iris,** which, no longer clinging to the corneo-scleral envelope, lies as a coronal sheet behind the cornea. Its muscles are disposed as a pupillary sphincter, encircling the pupillary rim, and a sheet of radiating fibres that forms the pupillary dilator. Before birth the pupil is occluded by vascular mesoderm, and even in later life fine strands of a 'persistent pupillary membrane' can often be seen. The complex developmental history of the eye yields a corresponding harvest of other congenital anomalies, and in the iris these readily provoke attention. Thus a sector-shaped gap or 'coloboma' is not uncommon, which may extend backwards to involve the ciliary body and choroid; or the iris may be totally absent ('aniridia'), or of a different colour from its fellow ('heterochromia'). In albinos the iris is translucent and pink, since its only remaining pigment is haemoglobin.

The **aqueous humour,** whose physiology is very similar to that of the cerebrospinal fluid, oozes from the capillaries of the iris and ciliary muscle, and circulates from the 'posterior chamber' (lying behind the iris) to reach the recesses of the 'anterior chamber' (between iris and cornea), whence it disperses into the episcleral veins via an encircling 'canal of Schlemm'.

The **lens** consists of a clear viscous matrix within a thin elastic capsule; and it lies in contact with the posterior surface of the iris suspended by its 'ligament' from the ciliary body. The ciliary muscle acts primarily as sphincter, so that, on contraction, it relaxes the suspensory ligament, and hence also the elastic lens capsule, with the result that the lens becomes more spherical, and thus focuses for near-vision.

Lining the inner surface of the choroid is the **retina,** with its rods and cones up against the choroidal surface, and the various cell relays running forwards and inwards, so that the fibres of the innermost 'ganglion cells' lie in contact with the vitreous surface. These fibres course (along with the retinal vessels) towards the optic nerve-head, or 'optic disc', and thence as the fibres of the optic nerve[1] back through the chiasma to their next relay in the lateral geniculate body. The fibres from the temporal half of the retina (carrying impulses from the nasal half of the visual field of that eye) come to lie laterally in the optic nerve, so that a lesion to the lateral side of the nerve will cause a loss of the nasal visual field. At the chiasma, the medial fibres cross over, and an interruption of the crossing fibres (as by a pituitary tumour) causes a corresponding bi-temporal hemianopia. Further back, a lesion of the right optic tract, radiations or occipital cortex will cause a left homonymous hemianopia (loss of the left half-field of each eye); with the upper quadrant of the field principally impaired when the lower fibres of tract, radiations or cortex are principally damaged and vice-versa.

The *GENERAL EXAMINATION* of the eye demands little beyond a good light, a magnifying lens ('loupe'), and an ophthalmoscope; and the principles of examination are really self-evident. One should start by noting the 'setting' of the two eyes,

[1] These fibres have no medullary sheath until they reach the optic nerve-head. Occasionally medullation transgresses a little onto the retinal surface, as a striking but harmless congenital anomaly (Fig. 57c, facing p. 65).

any asymmetry of their position, size or colour, particularly any difference in size of the palpebral aperture (as from a relative ptosis, or proptosis) or in size of the pupil. Then should follow a check of the pupil reactions to light—direct and consensual (from illumination of the fellow-eye) and to accommodation-convergence; and a check of the eye-movements, by fixing the patient's head with one hand and asking him to watch one's finger as it travels upward, downward, to left and to right (the relative positions of the two bright corneal light-reflections will betray an eye that lags in any particular direction of gaze). Then one turns to the individual eyes, checking in turn each of the structures from before backwards (lids, conjunctiva, cornea, iris and pupil, lens, and then with the ophthalmoscope,[1] the fundus). Finally, the intra-ocular pressure is checked by fluctuating the down-turned eye between one's two fore-fingers and contrasting its impressibility with that of its fellow or a normal eye (Fig. 41); and then the distance vision is assessed.

This **Visual Acuity** (Fig. 5) is normally tested by 'Snellen's types', at a distance of 6 metres (to exclude all but a negligible amount of accommodation). Vision is expressed as a fraction of the normal, the smallest letter normally visible without effort is thus '6/6'; if the patient can only see the letter twice its size, his visual acuity is '6/12'; while the largest letter usually displayed (10 times its size, and thus comfortably visible to the normal-sighted at 60 metres distance) designates a visual acuity of '6/60'. Still poorer vision is indicated by his capacity to count fingers ('C.F.'), see hand movements ('H.M.') and finally just

[1] *Notes on basic Technique.* Use right eye for right eye of patient and vice-versa, placing left hand on patient's forehead, with thumb elevating upper lid. Patient fixes eyes on object straight ahead. Surgeon holds Ophthalmoscope (without any lens interposed) up against his nose (keeping his other eye open if possible), gradually approaching patient at about 15° lateral to line of fixation, so that the patient's optic disc should be brought immediately into view (and promptly assessed, lest it is never seen again!). If it is out of focus, rotate into place increasingly strong concave lenses; if still out of of focus, consider lens or vitreous opacities. Then follow down the four vascular trunks looking for retinopathy; and finally check the macula (if elusive, ask the patient to look straight into the light).

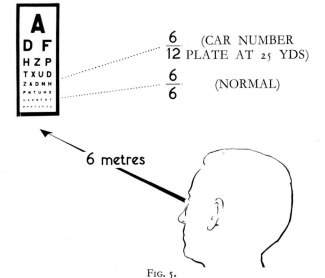

Fig. 5.
Testing visual acuity by Snellen's types.

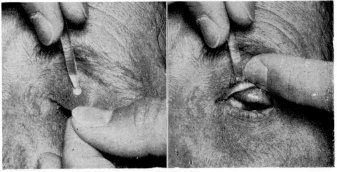

Fig. 6.
Eversion of the Upper Lid. (Wybar.)

to perceive light ('P.L.'). Near vision is similarly tested by a card bearing graded sizes of print.

Certain *SUPPLEMENTARY TESTS* are needed in special

cases. The under surface of the upper lid can easily be inspected by **everting the lid** over a finger or glass rod (Fig. 6); this is most easily done by standing behind the patient, who is told to look at the floor, and then pulling the upper lashes forwards and upwards, so that the lid is rolled over the upper edge of its

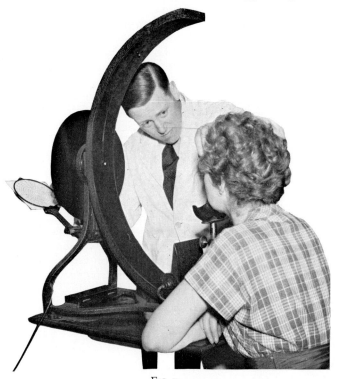

FIG. 7.
Technique of Perimetry, with the self-recording perimeter.
(Blaxter.)

tarsal plate which is meanwhile pressed backwards by the fore-finger of the other hand. The **visual fields** can be quickly assessed by the 'confrontation test', in which the patient closes one eye, looking straight with the other eye into the corresponding eye of the surgeon, and signals as soon as he can see the surgeon's fingers which are introduced in turn from the periphery in the four diagonal positions. But a more exact record is offered by the perimeter (Fig. 7) which charts the position where a small white target first becomes visible in each successive meridian, while the patient keeps his uncovered eye fixed on the 'hub' of the instrument (cf. charts, Figs. 56, 63, 64).

Colour-blindness is a curious hereditary defect found in about 8 per cent of men and 0.4 per cent of women, usually entailing a difficulty in differentiating red and green; it is readily tested by presenting a series of book-plates in which the different coloured spots spell out a number which will be specifically misinterpreted by the various colour-blind variants. **Night-blindness** is another hereditary defect, less readily tested, equally important in certain employments, and equally un-treatable.

Examination of the eyeball in *SMALL REFRACTORY CHILDREN* may require firm measures; the child should be wrapped tightly in a blanket, laid on a couch, with its head rigidly held between the assistant's hands. The eyelids can then be prised apart by simple 'retractors'. If the fundus also needs inspection, the wandering eye may have to be secured by conjunctival forceps after local or general anaesthesia.

CHAPTER II

THE EYELIDS, LACRIMAL AND ORBITAL TISSUES

THE eyelids are protective folds, covered by skin on the outside and a thin layer of conjunctiva beneath (this is the 'tarsal conjunctiva', as opposed to 'bulbar conjunctiva' where this same layer is continued over the surface of the sclera, and 'fornix conjunctiva', where these two layers meet in the recesses of the 'conjunctival sac'). The substance of the eyelid consists of two layers; anteriorly the Orbicularis Oculi muscle which closes the lid, and posteriorly a tarsal plate, the thickened wall of a row of 20–30 elongated sebaceous ('Meibomian') glands, which serves as a skeleton to the lid. Between these two layers lie the terminal fibres of the Levator Palpebrae Superioris muscle (Fig. 8).

The eyelid margin is divided longitudinally by a grey line marking the junction of skin and conjunctiva; along the anterior strip lie the eyelashes with sudorific and sebaceous glands at their roots, and posteriorly lie the openings of the Meibomian glands.

CONGENITAL MALFORMATIONS

Ptosis (a droop of the upper lid) calls for surgical correction if it is too unsightly, or in more extreme cases if it covers the pupil and interferes with vision; as ptosis is usually bilateral, such children may have to tilt their heads backwards in order to see beneath the drooping lids. Many operations have been proposed, but it is usually best simply to resect some of the levator palpebrae superioris muscle and of the upper tarsal plate.

Ptosis may also follow damage to the lid, levator muscle or its motor innervation (as in myasthenia gravis or tabes), or as a senile myasthenia when the lax tissues of old-age tend to sag.

Epicanthic folds are vertical pleats of skin between the
medial ends of the upper and lower lids which tend to overlap

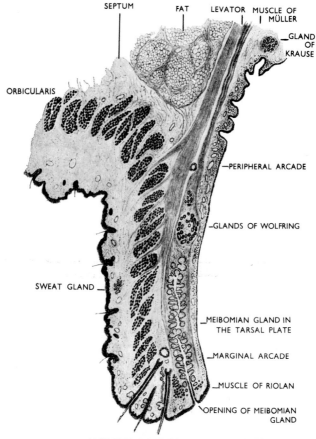

Fig. 8.
Vertical Section through the Upper Lid. (Wolff, *Anatomy of the Eye and Orbit.*)

the medial angle of the eye (Fig. 9). These are common in infants, where they often give the illusion of a convergent squint, and disappear when the nasal bones grow; occasionally they persist and require operative correction; and they are a normal feature of mongoloid races and 'mongolian' idiots.

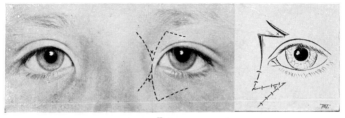

FIG. 9.

Epicanthic folds. On the left side, the skin incisions of Spaeth's operation are marked, and the triangular flaps are rotated as in the diagram alongside.

INFLAMMATION OF THE EYELIDS

Styes are localized infections of the glands of the lid margin. The more common 'external stye' (or 'Hordeolum'—Fig. 10)

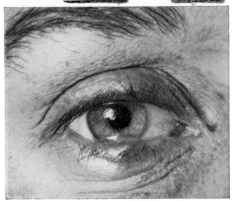

FIG. 10.
External Stye.

is a simple pyogenic infection of one of the glands at the lash-base, analogous to furuncles elsewhere; after a few days of painful induration, it normally discharges its bead of pus, and is gone. No treatment is necessary; heat is a mild palliative and doubtful expediter, and antibiotic ointment may prevent the emergent staphylococci from infecting another lash follicle farther down the line.

The 'internal stye' is a similar infection of one of the Meibomian glands. Since the gland-wall is tough, the pus rarely bursts through the skin or conjunctival surface, so that the inflammation is brought under control more slowly; and since the outlet of the gland has normally become blocked, its secretion combined with the inflammatory exudate distend the gland leaving a residual cyst—a **Meibomian cyst**—(Fig. 11), also

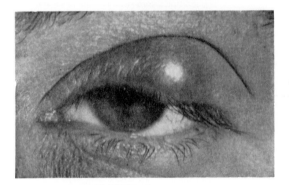

Fig. 11.
Meibomian Cyst.

known as 'Chalazion', since it feels like a hailstone embedded in the tarsal plate. These cysts are usually symptomless and may even develop insidiously, but, once established, they can only be dispersed surgically by incising vertically through the conjunctival surface and evacuating their mucinous content with a curette (Fig. 12).

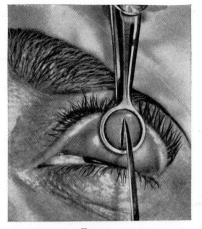

FIG. 12.
Evacuation of Meibomian Cyst.

A **Blepharitis** is a generalized infection of the margins of the eyelids, making the lid-margins look red, with a variable itchiness and an occasional discharge. This infection is notoriously persistent, and after some years the lashes often fall out or become distorted (such ingrowing lashes—'Trichiasis'—are liable to irritate and ulcerate the cornea). The milder form of blepharitis—'squamous blepharitis'—is essentially an outpost of dandruff from the scalp in seborrhoeic subjects, exhibiting similar scales clinging to the lashes, and provoking a similar variable irritation. The more severe 'ulcerative blepharitis' (Fig. 13) involves a staphylococcal infection on top of the seborrhoeic pityrosporon infection, and the lid margins become manifestly indurated and even ulcerated. Treatment must be long-sustained to be effective, as the infection is hard to eradicate. It entails (1) control of the scalp infection by frequent shampoos and anti-dandruff inunctions; (2) removal of all crusts and discharge from the lashes by an alkaline lotion, trimming the lashes if necessary; (3) drops or ointment containing a hydrocortisone and an antibiotic (as neomycin or chloramphenicol) to the lid margins at frequent intervals (1–2 hourly) for several weeks, and again at every relapse.

A seborrhoeic blepharitis is probably the commonest cause of all chronic eye discomforts, and this can nearly always be allayed simply by the use of topical steroids; but these must be prescribed with caution, as they carry the risk of exacerbating a dendritic corneal ulcer, or promoting a simple glaucoma (although the latter is rare before middle-age).

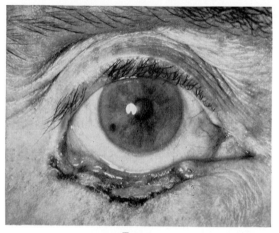

FIG. 13.
Ulcerative Blepharitis.

DISPLACEMENTS OF THE EYELIDS

The eyelids may become everted or inverted, and this may be due to *spasm* of the orbicularis (in infants this usually everts, and in adults usually inverts), *atony* of orbicularis (this correspondingly tends to invert in infants and evert in adults) or *scarring* (this everts if the skin is scarred—a 'cicatricial ectropion', as after burns of the face, and inverts if the tarsal conjunctiva is scarred—a 'cicatricial entropion', as in trachoma— Fig. 33). The common adult forms are thus a spastic entropion and an atonic ectropion.

Spastic Entropion (Fig. 14) is the product of persistent 'screwing up' and rubbing of the eyes, in irritable old people with irritable conjunctivae. A vicious circle develops, the lashes becoming inturned and causing more corneal and conjunctival irritation, with still further stimulus to entropion. Lubricants

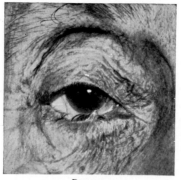

FIG. 14.
Spastic Entropion.

and sedatives may relieve, but surgery is usually needed, the simplest procedure being a 'skin-and-muscle operation', in which

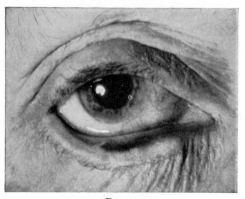

FIG. 15.
Atonic Ectropion.

a strip of skin and its underlying muscle are excised from the lower lid; and the resultant scarring, combined with the weakening of the orbicularis, usually suffices to prevent the entropion recurring.

Atonic Ectropion (Fig. 15) may be due to a flaccid orbicularis from a facial nerve palsy, or more commonly just a senile atony of the lower lid muscles which lets the lid droop away from the eyeball. A vicious circle again develops, since a stagnant pool of tears forms in the lower fornix, becomes infected, and causes a thickening of the inflamed conjunctiva which mechanically pushes the lid farther away, and increases the epiphora (= weeping) which is the prime symptom. Astringents may reduce the epiphora and antibiotics may reduce the infection, but an operation is again usually necessary, either to improve the lacrimal drainage by enlarging the punctum backwards into the stagnant pool (a 'three-snip operation') or as a plastic operation to tauten the lid.

TUMOURS AND DEGENERATIONS

Among benign tumours of the lids the most singular are **Xanthelasmata,** which are intradermal plaques of creamy xanthomatous deposits, generally symmetrical and sited at the medial ends of the upper or lower lids (Fig. 16). They are rarely

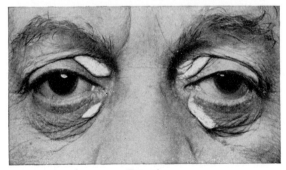

Fig. 16.
Xanthelasma.

related to any generalized lipoidosis, although they tend to arise in women of 'gallstone' diathesis; and they can always be excised if disfiguring. **Papillomata** are fairly common where conjunctiva and skin meet at the lid-margin, and may grow into horns several inches long. **Dermoid cysts** arise classically at the upper inner and outer angles of the orbit, while creamy 'dermolipomata' are often found astride the infant's corneo-scleral margin.

Of malignant tumours, **Rodent Ulcers** frequently arise (and carcinomas occasionally) at the lid-margin, and should be excised, or, if this would render plastic repair too clumsy, irradiated. **Carcinoma of the lacrimal gland** is much rarer, resembling in its structure and behaviour a mixed parotid tumour, since it generally starts as a benign adenoma, which, being loculated, is not easily removed completely, and recurrences often become malignant. In such cases it is best to excavate the entire orbital contents (an 'exenteration').

Pingueculae and **Pterygia** are fairly common degenerative growths on the front of the eye which may be included here. A Pinguecula is a fatty deposit under the conjunctiva which is often most arresting when it fails to share in any coincident conjunctival congestion; a Pterygium is a wing-shaped fold of

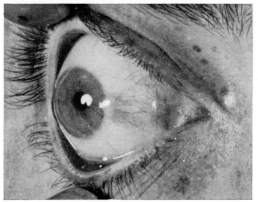

FIG. 17.
Pterygium.

conjunctiva that gradually transgresses onto the cornea, and may even reach the central area and impair vision (Fig. 17). Both are symptomless and symmetrical, involve only the medial and lateral sides, and tend to occur after a life of exposure to the elements; and both of them can readily be excised, although the resultant scar may yield little cosmetic improvement. The Pterygium may also need excision if it threatens the sight, and various techniques are employed to try and prevent recurrence. Other purely corneal degenerations include the familiar **arcus senilis** (a white encircling ring, about 1 mm. within the corneal margin) which affects only the periphery, and therefore never damages sight; and the **familial dystrophies**, which affect the central area, and distort the vision. The latter can readily be replaced by a corneal graft.

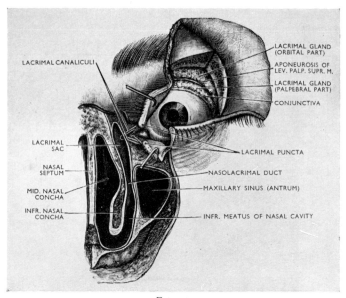

Fig. 18.
The Anatomy of the Lacrimal Apparatus. (Gray's *Anatomy*.)

DACRYOCYSTITIS

The lacrimal sac, lying in a fossa in the lacrimal bone, collects the tears from the two narrow canaliculi and transmits them downwards through the nasolacrimal duct into the lower meatus of the nasal cavity (Fig. 18). Epiphora may be the legacy of a block at the punctum (sometimes it is plugged by a detached eye-lash) or in the canaliculus (as from a laceration of the lid margin, or the not infrequent cheesy agglomerations of streptothrix), or else simply by an eversion of the lid margin (ectropion). More usually it follows an obstruction of the nasolacrimal duct, either as a result of a sac infection (dacryocystitis) or in the infant from a failure in canalization (in which case a secondary dacryocystitis soon follows).

Acute Dacryocystitis is usually induced by a pneumococcus which ascends from the nasopharynx, and it is evidenced by a tender induration at the medial angle of the eye. Pus may rupture through the skin forming a fistula, but more usually it resolves (especially when allayed by local heat and systemic antibiotics), to leave a chronic dacryocystitis with a blocked nasolacrimal duct, and sometimes a visibly distended 'mucocele' of the sac; more often a chronic dacryocystitis develops without antecedent acute phase, particularly in elderly women. The cardinal symp-

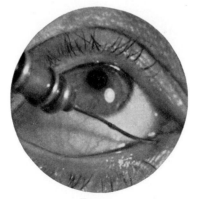

FIG. 19.
Syringing the Lacrimal Sac.

tom of chronic dacryocystitis is epiphora, and the overflowing tears may be augmented by the discharge from a chronic conjunctivitis, which has been provoked by regurgitation of pus along the lacrimal canaliculi.

The treatment of this epiphora entails (1) syringing of saline through the lower canaliculus (Fig. 19); this shows whether there is a nasolacrimal duct obstruction, and in the early stages may in fact clear the blocked passage; (2) Astringent drops or lotions, such as Zinc Sulphate ½ per cent, to reduce the watering; (3) Operation, if the epiphora is sufficiently troublesome and has not yielded to several syringings; ideally this should be a 'dacryocystorhinostomy' (Fig. 20), fashioning a new stoma between the

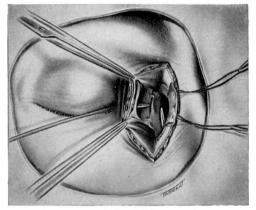

FIG. 20.

Dacryocystorhinostomy. The posterior flaps of the medial sac wall and nasal mucosa have been sutured together. Probes have been inserted through the canaliculus and the nose, to demonstrate the reconstituted passage. (Lyle.)

sac and the middle nasal meatus, but in the old and debile, especially where regurgitation of pus is the main trouble, a 'dacryocystectomy' may suffice to ease the symptoms by simply removing the source of conjunctival re-infection; (4) Probing the nasolacrimal duct is of value only in the absence of established infection—i.e. when the infantile duct has failed to canalize; such cases are usually cured by toilet and antibiotic drops alone, but probing is generally advised if the blockage persists for several months; (5) Finally, epiphora may be relieved, when the lacrimal outlet cannot be re-established, by reducing the production of tears, either by excising or by injecting alcohol into the lacrimal gland (at the outer upper angle of the orbit).

EXOPHTHALMOS

Any lesion within the unyielding bony walls of the orbit tends to push the eyeball forwards and present as an exophthalmos (or 'proptosis', which strictly means a protrusion of the lids as well). Where the pressure is exerted from directly behind the eye (as from a haemorrhage, inflammation or tumour within the cone of the four rectus muscles) the eye is pushed directly forwards, but an eccentric pressure (as from a periostitis or lacrimal gland tumour) will deviate the eyeball and present with diplopia, unless the sight has already been destroyed.

Carotico-cavernous Fistula, due to trauma or spontaneous rupture of a carotid aneurysm into the enveloping cavernous sinus, permits a reflux of arterial blood under pressure into the orbital veins. It presents classically as a 'pulsating exophthalmos', and though the systolic pulsations may be barely visible, they are audible both to the auscultating surgeon and to the patient as an alarming noise, likened to the buzz of a bluebottle within a paper bag or the rush of a millstream. The conjunctival vessels are visibly engorged, and both lids and conjunctivae may be very oedematous; these same signs are usually present, but less well-marked, on the other side (via the connecting intercavernous sinuses). The condition is generally stationary, but the initial pain recedes, and in the absence of ocular complications the initially lowered vision may also slowly improve. Radical treatment entails ligation of the common carotid or (if this fails) internal carotid artery, both yielding about a 50 per cent cure and an appreciable mortality rate.

Orbital Cellulitis (Fig. 21), generally deriving from an adjacent sinusitis, is fairly common, and grave because of the risk of damage to the eye or of extension back to the meninges. The eyeball protrudes and becomes immobile, and the sight may be extinguished by pressure on the optic nerve (although a pallor of the optic disc will not be visible for some weeks, and the fundus at first shows only a venous engorgement); pain is often severe until pus is evacuated, but prompt treatment with systemic antibiotics usually permits resolution without any recourse to operative drainage.

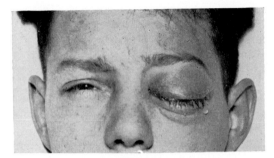

FIG. 21.

Acute Orbital Cellulitis, following an acute sinusitis, and exhibiting proptosis with oedema of lids and conjunctiva.

Cavernous Sinus Thrombosis may be the drastic sequel to orbital cellulitis or may follow some simple pyogenic infection such as a furuncle that has drained via the angular vein into the cavernous sinus. The signs and symptoms are largely an aggravation of those of an orbital cellulitis, but the degree of pain, extreme venous congestion and bilaterality are usually diagnostic; in any event the same treatment obtains, supplemented by anticoagulants to prevent extensions of the septic clot.

Dysthyroid Exophthalmos—There are two main types of ophthalmic manifestation in thyroid disease, mild and severe, the one merging imperceptibly into the other.

The mild type (Fig. 22) occurs classically in patients with Grave's disease and is seen most commonly in women aged

20–50, along with the general signs of thyrotoxicosis (tremor, sweating, wasting and tachycardia). Lid-retraction and lid-lag are often marked and result in a prominent stare; there may, in addition, be a mild degree of proptosis. The systemic treatment

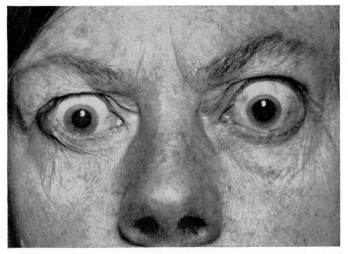

FIG. 22.

Mild Dysthyroid Exophthalmos (Graves's disease) lateral tarsorrhaphy has been performed on the R. side,

is that of the underlying hyperthyroidism, and includes sedatives, antithyroid drugs, radio-active iodine and thyroidectomy. The ocular changes rarely merit attention, but a small lateral tarsorrhaphy may be cosmetically helpful, while lid retraction sometimes responds to guanethidine eyedrops indicating its probable origin from overactivity of the sympathetic nervous system.

The severe type (Fig. 23) is much less common and affects the sexes equally, at an average age of 50. It often follows the treatment of hyperthyroidism and the patient may show under- or over-activity of the gland. This condition is not clearly understood but it is apparently caused by an exophthalmos-producing

C

substance, probably a gamma globulin but possibly a product of the pituitary gland. The systemic signs are usually slight and the ocular signs predominate, with a gross and irreducible exophthalmos, frequently leading to corneal ulceration, a marked ophthalmoplegia especially of upward movement and even preceding the exophthalmos, and a marked oedema of lids and conjunctivae. These changes are due to an infiltration and oedema with subsequent fibrosis of the muscles themselves, and to a lesser extent of the other orbital tissues. Systemic treatment of the underlying thyroid condition is neither very efficacious nor very necessary since the condition is self-limiting, but the grave risk of corneal damage or strangulation of the optic nerve generally calls for urgent treatment. Some cases respond dramatically to large doses of systemic steroids, but failing this a wide tarsorrhaphy or even an orbital decompression may be necessary.

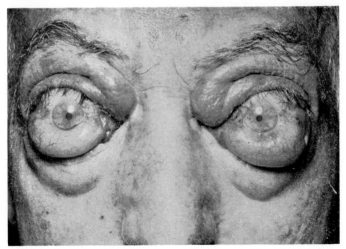

FIG. 23.
Severe Dysthyroid Exophthalmos; with ophthalmoplegia and oedema.

CHAPTER III

SQUINT

SQUINT (or 'Strabismus') means a deviation of the eyes[1] so that their axes are no longer parallel, but excluding the normal convergence that accompanies near-vision. Deviations may be in any direction, but are most commonly horizontal (convergent or divergent). Such a deviation of the visual axes is obvious if the squint is gross; but small degrees of squint can be recognised from the asymmetrical positions of the bright corneal light-reflections relative to their respective pupil margins, and confirmed by covering each eye in turn, and noting whether a perceptible movement is made by either eye to assume fixation, when its fellow-eye is occluded.

The eyes are kept parallel by a complicated conditioned reflex, acquired during the first few years of life in the interests of single vision; this reflex is consolidated when the child learns to fuse the two superimposed images (from either eye) and finally to appreciate stereoscopic vision. A squint may arise from damage to the motor-apparatus that rotates the eye (a *paralytic squint*) or else to the sensory apparatus that transmits the images for fusion (e.g. a poor-sighted eye from any cause) or to the central component of the reflex arc (e.g. mental deficiency, psychic disturbance, or, most commonly of all, some impediment, whose exact cause is unknown); the last two result in a *concomitant squint* in which the visual axes deviate at a constant angle irrespective of the direction of gaze.

PARALYTIC SQUINT

Signs and Symptoms—The affected eye will have *limited movement* in the direction of the action of the paralysed muscle; the *angle*

---

[1] The word 'squint' is sometimes carelessly and erroneously used to signify a half-closure of the eyes or the inspection of objects at a very close range.

of deviation will thus be greatest in that direction, and the *double-vision* that results will similarly be greatest in that same direction.

The secondary signs include an *alteration of posture*: thus a paralysed left lateral rectus will cause an increasing squint and increasing double-vision ('diplopia') on looking to the left, but on looking to the right the left lateral rectus will not be needed, and the visual axes will become parallel; the patient thus learns to avoid diplopia by turning his head to the left and looking out of the right-hand corner of his eyes.   Similarly a tilt of the head laterally or forwards (Fig. 24) may compensate for

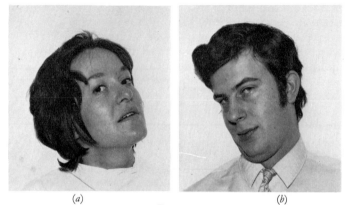

(*a*)   (*b*)

Fig. 24.

Ocular torticollis. Examples of compensating postures: (a) Face turned to L., head tilted to R., chin elevated—to compensate for Left Supr. Rectus palsy; (b) Face turned to R., head tilted to R., chin depressed—to compensate for Left Supr. Oblique palsy.

weakness of one of the vertically-acting muscles (requiring differentiation from the other forms of torticollis).

Paralysis of the lateral and medial recti produces a simple horizontal deviation of the eyes and horizontal diplopia; the line of action of the other extra-ocular muscles is more complex (Fig. 25). The superior and inferior recti both take origin at the orbital apex which is well medial to the eyeball's centre of rotation, and thus both tend to adduct the eye, as well as elevating and depressing it respectively; only when the eye is directed laterally (*abducted*) so that it lies along the axis of these rectus muscles do the latter act as pure elevators or depressors; and when the eye is *adducted*, so that it is directed almost perpendicular to their axis, these rectus muscles act almost entirely as adductors (Fig. 26). Similarly the two oblique muscles have a secondary effect of abducting, which is most marked when the eyes are already abducted; while they act almost entirely as elevators (the

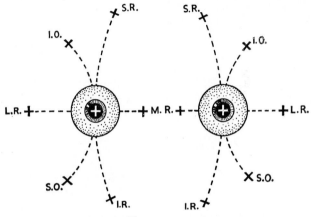

Fig. 25.

The line of action of the individual extra-ocular muscles, showing also their torsional effects, and indicating the various contralateral synergists (S.R.+ I.O. (I.R.+S O.) M.R.+L.R.).

inferior obliques) and depressors (the superior obliques) when the eye is adducted and lies nearly along their line of action— running from the anteromedial corners of the orbit to insert at the back of the eye on its outer aspect (Fig. 26). These vertical muscles thus act in concert, the superior rectus and inferior oblique collaborating to elevate the eye (neutralizing each other's secondary effects of abduction and adduction), while the superior and inferior recti will both assist the medial rectus in adducting the eye, and neutralizing each other's vertical pull. A further complication of these four vertically-acting muscles is their tertiary effect in 'torsion'—rolling the eye about an antero-posterior axis (thus the superior rectus rolls the top of the eye over towards the nose, causing an 'intorsion'); these effects are similarly neutralized by the collaboration of different muscles in each ocular movement, aided by the synergistic muscles of the fellow eye.

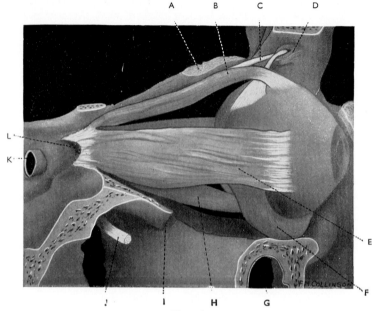

FIG. 26.

Anatomy of the extra-ocular muscles from the lateral aspect. (A) Levator Palpebrae Superioris Muscle; (B) Superior Rectus Muscle; (C) Superior Oblique Muscle; (D) Pulley; (E) Lateral Rectus Muscle; (F) Inferior Oblique Muscle; (G) Maxillary Antrum; (H) Inferior Rectus Muscle; (I) Inferior Orbital Fissure; (J) Maxillary Nerve (Vb); (K) Internal Carotid Artery; (L) Optic Foramen. (Wolff, *Anatomy of the Eye and Orbit.*)

Assessment—The limitation of movement may be obvious (Fig. 27). The diplopia is usually of sudden onset, and disappears on covering either eye; and the more blurred and more displaced image will belong to the affected eye. The palsied muscles can be

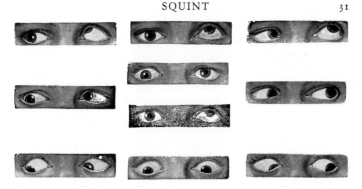

FIG. 27.

Deviation of the eyes in paralysis of the R. Superior rectus, in each of the nine cardinal directions of gaze. The two central pictures show the deviation on looking straight ahead, the upper one when the left eye is fixing, and the lower one when the right eye is fixing. (Duke-Elder, *Textbook of Ophthalmology*.)

identified by noting in which of the nine positions of gaze the diplopia is worst, and the eye from which the respective images are derived can be distinguished by the wearing of different coloured goggles (Fig. 28).

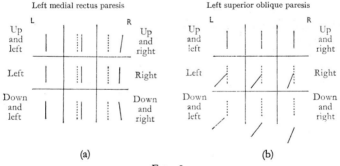

FIG. 28.

The assessment of Diplopia by charting the doubled images, in the case of paresis of (a) left medial rectus, and (b) left superior oblique. The patient wears a red glass in front of the right eye, and the dotted line shows the position of this right-eye's image. (After Lyle and Jackson.)

Aetiology—Any cause of nerve or muscle damage may be responsible. The common causes include: Trauma (to brain or orbit), vascular disease (e.g. aneurysm of circle of Willis, intra-orbital or intra-cranial haemorrhage, or thrombosis of the nutrient vessels to the individual nerves), neuritis (e.g. disseminated sclerosis or syphilis), metabolic (e.g. dysthyroid exophthalmos), cerebral tumour, etc.

Treatment—Any evident underlying disease must first have attention. The diplopia may then be relieved—most simply by occluding the deviating eye (e.g. by tissue-paper gummed on its spectacle lens); while in an established paralysis surgery to the extra-ocular muscles can at least render the eyes straight when looking directly forwards, and discordant eye movements can then be largely avoided by movement of the head rather than the eyes.

CONCOMITANT SQUINT

Here the eyes adopt an abnormal position in relation to one another—usually of convergence, but the complicated yoking of the eye movements (by reciprocal innervation) serves to keep this angle of deviation constant in all directions of gaze. Such a concomitant squint normally develops during the first few years of life, before the reflex of binocular vision has had time to become established; and, when it has not been induced early from some organic impediment to vision (e.g. a congenital cataract), it is often precipitated when illness or emotional travail so depletes the child's energies that he can no longer make the subconscious effort to keep the eyes straight. In such cases the infant's eyes generally exhibit their natural tendency to converge; (infants are long-sighted, and this entails an excess of accommodation; as the 'near-reflex' is a synkinesis involving accommodation, convergence and pupillary constriction, each one of these movements tends automatically to induce the other two).

Infants can quickly learn to suppress the vision of such a squinting eye, to avoid the diplopia that such a deviation must first induce; and if this suppression is maintained for several years, it may become impossible to counteract, so that the eye remains permanently poor-sighted—an *'amblyopia'*, or, more familiarly, a 'lazy eye'. Sometimes the child learns to suppress the vision of either eye at will, so that both eyes retain good vision but cannot be used in unison—an 'alternating concomitant convergent squint'. As age advances there is an increasing tendency for the eyes to diverge, thus convergent concomitant squints do tend to straighten later (a 'natural cure'), although usually at the expense of a half-blinded amblyopic eye; while eyes blinded in adult life similarly tend to swing outwards sooner or later.

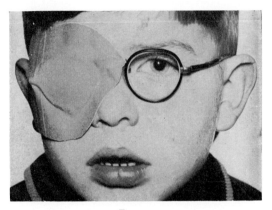

FIG. 29.

Occlusion of the better-seeing eye in squint. The simplest method is by fixing two layers of Elastoplast over the spectacle lens, and trimming this to fit the patient's face.

Treatment—The first essential is to prevent the development of amblyopia before it is too late, in most cases this is done by *occluding* the better-seeing eye (Fig. 29), and so forcing the child to use the squinting eye; this is usually successful before the age of 7 and rarely after the age of 10. The underlying tendency to converge must then be neutralized by correcting any hypermetropia with appropriate convex *spectacles* (infants are very rarely myopic, but in such cases there will be a corresponding tendency to develop a divergent squint). If a marked squint persists in spite of correct glasses and the prevention of amblyopia, an *operation* is usually indicated to re-align the squinting eye (Fig. 30); this normally entails the reinsertion of the medial rectus tendon farther back on the globe (a 'recession') and an equivalent shortening of the lateral rectus tendon (a 'resection'). Operation is usually advised about the age of 5, by which time the child can also collaborate in *orthoptic exercises*. These are sensory

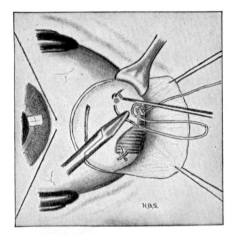

FIG. 30.

Operation for Squint. Recession of the R. medial rectus. Two sutures hold apart the edges of the conjuctival incision, and two 'whip' sutures unite the upper and lower margins of the muscle to the sclera some 5 mm. behind the line of its former (severed) insertion. (Stallard, *Eye Surgery*.)

exercises that help the eyes to build up their fusion and ultimately their stereoscopic vision (and not exercises for the eye-muscles); such exercises will rarely cure a squint, but the presence of full binocular vision will always help to keep straight those eyes which spectacles or operation have brought into rough alignment. Squinting eyes can always be brought straight by operation at any age for cosmetic effect, but they may well drift out of alignment later, as there will be no further development of binocular vision and no significant return of vision in an amblyopic eye over the age of 10. Because of the rapid decline of the child's capacity to recover suppressed vision and to achieve full binocularity, all squinting children should be referred for specialist advice as soon as the squint is noted.

LATENT SQUINT—Signifies a tendency to squint which has usually developed after the child has acquired enough binocular vision to hold the eyes normally in alignment, and only when the objects presented to the two eyes are different, or fatigue prevails, does a concomitant squint become manifest. Such latent squints can very occasionally be relieved by prismatic glasses, sometimes they even need an operative correction, but generally they cause no symptoms and require no active treatment. A small degree of horizontal latent squint is indeed present in most healthy eyes.

NYSTAGMUS—These oscillations of the eyes may be ocular or labyrinthine-cerebellar in origin.

The *ocular nystagmus* has regular pendulum-like movements, which are exaggerated on looking to either side; the movements are generally horizontal, but may have a vertical or rotatory component. It may derive from some manifest impediment to macular fixation (as in albinos), as a 'miner's nystagmus' where the illumination is too poor to allow the macular cones to function, or as a congenital lapse in apparently healthy eyes (but which have a corresponding lowering of their central vision in consequence).

The *labyrinthine-cerebellar* nystagmus has movements that show a slow drift in one direction and a fast correcting jerk back again, the drift generally being towards the side of the lesion (e.g. middle-ear damage, acoustic neuroma), and the movements are usually exaggerated on looking in the opposite direction.

A rather indefinite, 'wobbling', nystagmus is particularly common in disseminated sclerosis.

CHAPTER IV

THE PAINFUL RED EYE

THERE are three main causes of the painful red eye: Inflammation of the outer eye (**acute conjunctivitis**), inflammation of the inner eye (**acute iritis**), and the congested, tense eyeball due to a sudden blockage of aqueous outflow (**acute glaucoma**). A knowledge of their differential diagnosis is consequently of extreme importance since the majority of eye affections demanding urgent treatment fall into one of these three categories. A fourth major cause of painful red eyes should properly be added to this list—an **acute keratitis** (which generally presents as the familiar 'corneal ulcer'); and, since the cornea is the gateway between the outer and inner eyes, the symptoms, signs and treatment of acute keratitis are correspondingly a combination of those of an acute conjunctivitis and an acute iritis.

ACUTE CONJUNCTIVITIS

SIGNS AND SYMPTOMS

1. *Injection*—this is a generalized 'conjunctival injection', equally manifest in the tarsal conjunctiva which lines the posterior surface of the eyelids (unlike the purely 'circumcorneal injection' of acute iritis and acute glaucoma) (Fig. 31).

2. *Discharge*—this is purulent, mucopurulent or catarrhal, according to severity of infection; most noticeable on waking, when the lids are often glued together.

3. *Discomfort*—this is a grittiness rather than a pain, primarily caused by the rubbing together of the congested bulbar and lid conjunctivae with every movement of the eyelids.

4. *Photophobia*—so mild that it can be relieved by dark glasses.

AETIOLOGICAL TYPES

The common catarrhal conjunctivitis is usually due to *Staph. aureus*; the rarer severe bout is often due to *Pneumococcus*. Less common types include 'Epidemic pink-eye' due to *Koch-Weeks bacillus*, and 'Angular Conjunctivitis' due to *Morax-Axenfield bacillus* (affecting the outer and inner angles of the eye); both

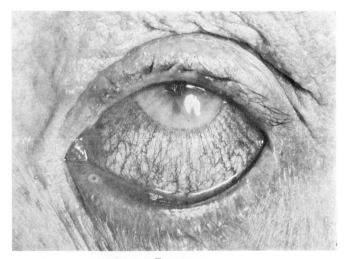

FIG. 31.
Acute Infective Conjunctivitis, with slight secondary ectropion and pouting of the lacrimal punctum.

the latter are small Haemophilus bacilli. Other forms are due to different *viruses* (such as 'inclusion body conjunctivitis'). The healthy conjunctiva often harbours Staphylococcus albus and Corynebacterium xerosis.

The forms of acute conjunctivitis essentially resemble a nasal catarrh; they usually subside in a week without lasting damage, and may be allayed by treatment.

There remain two serious conjunctival infections that often lead to blindness, both now rarely seen in England:

Ophthalmia neonatorum is a severe purulent conjunctivitis, (Fig. 32) contracted at birth from a *gonococcal* infection of the maternal passages. Formerly a cause of widespread blindness (from secondary corneal ulceration), it has now become rare since the general adoption of Crédé's prophylactic drops (1–2 per cent silver nitrate, instilled into the eye of every new-born baby); although nowadays these drops can safely be omitted, as long as subsequent medical supervision is ensured (for once recognized, gonococcal conjunctivitis now yields promptly to intensive penicillin applications or sulphonamides by mouth). Any eye discharge within 3 weeks of birth is a notifiable disease, although such a discharge is generally due to a viral infection, and free from danger.

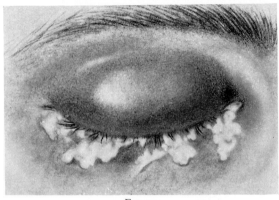

FIG. 32.

Acute Purulent Conjunctivitis. (Gonococcal 'Ophthalmia neonatorum'.)

Trachoma is a viral conjunctivitis, in which the organism, although morphologically similar to the other virus pathogens of the conjunctiva, can invade the underlying tissues. The sight is damaged by the secondary scarring of the cornea; initially this scarring follows a direct infection of the cornea, but it is also provoked in the later stages when cicatrization of the tarsal plate has induced an ectropion (leading to a neurotrophic keratitis from exposure) or an entropion (with inturned lashes abrading the cornea)—(Fig. 33, and see p. 16). Lymphoid hyperplasia is a characteristic of most viral conjunctivites, and the resultant follicles are especially apparent in trachoma, where they may

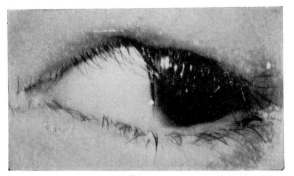

FIG. 33.

Late Trachoma. Cicatricial entropion of the upper lid with inturned lashes. (Scheie.)

cover the under surfaces of the tarsal plates, 1–3 mm. in diameter (Fig. 34). Trachoma has been endemic since pre-history in the Middle East, and sporadic in most other countries of the world with the striking and almost universal exception of the British

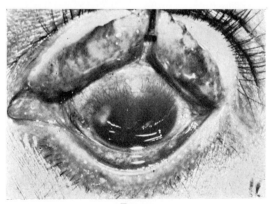

FIG. 34.

Early Trachoma. The upper tarsal conjunctiva is grossly thickened and covered in follicles, while a vascularized infiltrate ('pannus') is extending down over the upper cornea. (Scheie.)

Commonwealth; devastating outbreaks have followed in the wake of most invading armies that reached the Middle East (Crusades, Napoleonic wars) or set out from there (Mohammedan invasions). The virus is just within the range of antibiotic and sulphonamide therapy, which will also control any secondary bacterial infection, otherwise the treatment has consisted since early Classical times in repeated cautery of the everted conjunctivae with a crystal of copper sulphate ('the Blue Stone Stick').

ALLERGIC CONJUNCTIVITIS

The Conjunctiva often becomes hypersensitive to a miscellany or irritants. Some of these, such as the drugs (especially atropine and penicillin) or the cosmetics with which it is belaboured, principally effect the eyelids, causing eczema and oedema (Fig. 35). Other exogenous allergens, such as pollens, cause an extreme congestion and watering of the conjunctival and nasal

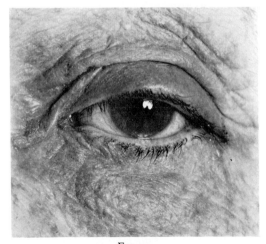

FIG. 35.
'Atropine Irritation.'
Allergic dermato-conjunctivitis due to atropine-sensitivity.

mucosa, as in **Hay fever**. Allergy from pollens may also be chronic and seasonal, as in **Spring catarrh**, characterised by flat-topped, translucent papules, mainly over the tarsal conjunctiva (Fig. 36).

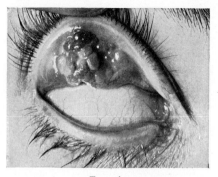

FIG. 36.

'Spring Catarrh.' Flat-topped papillae on the upper tarsal conjunctiva.

Endogenous allergens, such as tuberculo-protein, may pro-voke a **Phlyctenular conjunctivitis,** commonly seen in poorly nourished children before the last war, but now rare. This is characterized by subconjunctival aggregations of lymphocytes which appear as 'phlyctens', 1–2 mm. in diameter, and yellowish in contrast to the surrounding engorgement, which occasionally transgress onto the cornea, producing corneal ulcers (Fig. 37).

Conjunctival allergies usually respond specifically to treatment with drops of corticosteroids or anti-histamines (as Otrivine-Antistin), and can generally be allayed by astringents; desensi-tization is rarely applicable.

TREATMENT OF CONJUNCTIVITIS

1. *Remove discharge by irrigation with saline* (Fig. 38). If there is no discharge, irrigation is unnecessary but may be comforting.

D

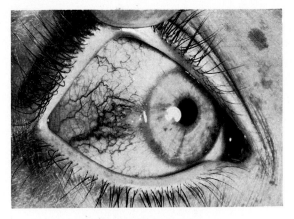

FIG. 37.

Phlyctenular Kerato-conjunctivitis with yellowish aggregations of leucocytes on the conjunctiva and encroaching onto the cornea.

2. *Bactericidal applications.* These must be given every hour or two to be of value. Penicillin is generally effective (10,000 U/ml.), but an increasing number of resistant strains and increasing incidence of skin-sensitivity often give preference at any rate with adults to chloramphenicol, which has a wide antibiotic spectrum, is stable and relatively cheap. Other antibiotic drops are indicated for resistant strains, such as tetracycline, streptomycin (Gram neg. bacilli), polymyxin (Ps. aeruginosa). Topical sulphonamides are rarely indicated, but sulphacetamide ('Albucid') is popular and of limited value.

3. *Symptomatic treatment.* Dark-glasses will allay the mild photophobia, but an eye-pad should be avoided since it may retain the discharge and incubate the pathogens. Lubricant drops as methyl cellulose (1 per cent) may relieve the 'grittiness', or the lubricant may be provided in the form of an ointment vehicle for the antibiotic agent.

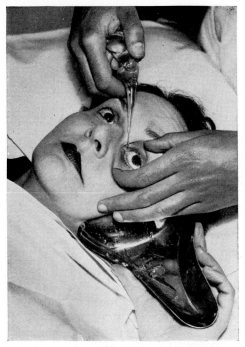

Fig. 38.

Irrigation of the Conjunctiva with an undine.

4. *Astringent applications.* Solutions of metallic salts will decongest and dry an inflamed eye, and relieve the feeling of heaviness and irritability. They are particularly useful where the inflammation is due to allergy, external irritants (smoke, ultra-violet light, etc.), or when the eye remains red after the infection has been cleared by antibiotic treatment. Zinc sulphate ($\frac{1}{4}$–$\frac{1}{2}$ per cent drops or lotion) or silver proteinate drops are usually advised; but where there is an allergic factor, corticosteroid drops are most effective (although used with caution—see p. 16).

ACUTE IRITIS

The iris, ciliary body and choroid form a continuous sheet along the inner wall of corneo-sclera, known as the 'uveal tract', and although each component is to some extent involved in any intra-ocular inflammation, the clinical picture of uveitis varies with the main site of its impact. When the burden falls on the anterior uvea (an 'iritis' or an 'irido-cyclitis') the eye becomes *painful* from oedema and from spasm of the iris and ciliary muscles, and *red* from engorgement of the adjacent circum-corneal vessels which are connected through the sclera with the vessels of the iris root. A 'choroiditis' is correspondingly pain-less, free from any visible congestion on the front of the eye, and presents simply with an *impairment of vision* (p. 69).

SIGNS AND SYMPTOMS

1. Engorgement of the episcleral vessels overlying the iris root, as a 'ciliary' or **'circumcorneal injection'** (Fig. 39). This differs from a 'conjunctival injection' (in which vessels are en-gorged evenly over the whole conjunctival surface—'tarsal' as well as 'bulbar') qualitatively as well as geographically, since these deeper episcleral vessels seem less discrete through the overlying conjunctiva (the term 'ciliary flush' is thus sometimes used), and the colour is a brick-red rather than pink (it becomes purple when a venous stasis rather than an inflammatory injection is responsible, as in the ciliary injection of an acute glaucoma).

2. **Contraction of the pupil,** to which the reflex spasm of the sphincter and the distension of the iris with blood both con-tribute.

3. Inflammatory **exudation** into the anterior chamber. Pus cells can always be discerned with the corneal microscope as a pathognomonic sign, and these may be so profuse that they gravitate to form an obvious fluid-level at the bottom of the anterior chamber, known as a **hypopyon** (Figs. 44 and 46). They also adhere to the back of the cornea forming clumps

Fig. 39 (*see page* 45).

Acute Iritis. Intense ciliary injection, and festooned pupil from the posterior synechiae which had formed before atropine was instilled.

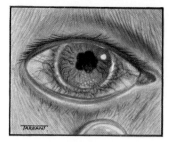

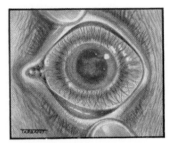

Fig. 42 (*see page* 50).

Acute Glaucoma. ('Primary Congestive Glaucoma.') Dusky ciliary injection, oval, dilated pupil and corneal haze.

Fig. 49 (*see page* 57).

Episcleritis. (Gifford's *Textbook of Ophthalmology*.)

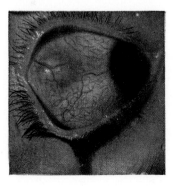

which are often visible macroscopically, and known as **keratic precipitates,** or more familiarly 'K.P.' (Fig. 40). This exudate causes a proportionate **blurring of vision,** especially when it also passes from the ciliary body into the vitreous (whence it is less readily dispersed).

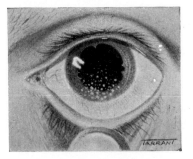

FIG. 40.
Keratic Precipitates.

4. Adhesions between iris and the anterior lens surface with which it is normally in contact. These are known as **'posterior synechiae',** as opposed to the rare anterior synechiae between iris and cornea, which can arise if the aqueous escapes through a perforating corneal wound or ulcer. Such posterior synechiae are often rendered obvious when the therapeutic atropine drops cause a festooning of the pupil, which dilates only between those points where its margin is already bound-down to the lens (Figs. 39 and 40). Should the whole pupillary margin become adherent, the aqueous, which oozes (mainly by diffusion) from the anterior surface of the iris and the ciliary body, cannot pass forwards through the pupil to reach its exit into the canal of Schlemm; and the iris may then become ballooned forward (an 'iris bombé'), and the intra-ocular pressure will rise (a 'secondary glaucoma').

5. The eyeball is **tender** and **painful;** this pain is constant, and does not cease when the eyelids are stilled, and may thus

keep the patient awake at night, unlike the simple irritation provoked by a conjunctivitis.

6. **Photophobia.** Light seems positively hurtful to the eye, unlike the mild light-sensitivity from a conjunctivitis which dark glasses will normally allay, and the lids may be difficult to open ('blepharospasm'); this is generally accompanied by a little reflex lacrimation (unlike the manifest inflammatory discharge of an acute conjunctivitis).

Acute iritis tends to last for weeks or even months, relapses being common, and leaving a proportionate amount of permanent visual damage. Sometimes the iritis is chronic, with little pain and injection, but the sight is insidiously reduced by the exudate, especially when this permeates behind the lens into the vitreous cavity. Complications include: **secondary glaucoma,** where the exudate or adhesions impede drainage of the aqueous, and **secondary cataract** through impairment of lens nutrition.

AETIOLOGICAL TYPES OF ACUTE IRITIS

Iritis (and uveitis generally) is occasionally caused by *exogenous* infection, gaining admission through perforating wounds of the eyeball or corneal ulcers, and leading to a purulent 'endophthalmitis', which becomes a 'panophthalmitis' if the outer coats have been invaded.

The large majority of cases of iritis are *endogenous*, and the cause is generally unknown; over the last fifty years these have been attributed in turn to syphilis, tuberculosis, focal sepsis (especially teeth), allergy, virus disease, auto-immunity and metabolic upset. A small percentage seem indeed to be due to each of these groups, as well as a variety of rarer affections (as ankylosing spondylitis, brucellosis, sarcoidosis, toxoplasmosis, gonorrhoea), but the genesis of the majority remains obscure. In investigating such cases, it is thus usual to exclude a positive Wassermann reaction, radiographic evidence of spondylitis or of infective foci in teeth, sinuses and chest, and possibly perform a Mantoux test, toxoplasmosis test and blood analysis.

Sympathetic Ophthalmitis is a specific form of iritis (or, more correctly, of uveitis), which generally follows perforating wounds near the corneo-scleral junction, including operations as for cataract, and which involves the other eye some weeks later, and is so persistent that it may render both eyes almost blind. It very rarely occurs within three weeks after the initiating injury, but any traumatic iritis which is not subsiding after such an interval is dangerous, and such an eye may even require excision to prevent the risk of involving its fellow. In treatment, corticosteroids are of especial benefit.

TREATMENT OF ACUTE IRITIS

1. **Corticosteroids,** which simply inhibit the inflammatory response, are of enormous value in allaying any uveitis, except in the very rare case where there is a frank infective agent, for such uveites are essentially self-limiting, and both the ultimate damage and the degree of pain that is provoked are largely proportional to the intensity of the inflammatory reaction. Patients with this form of anterior uveitis should receive as much steroid as is necessary to keep the eye quiet; topical application is of course free of any systemic side-effects as well as the expense of systemic steroid therapy. So drops or ointment ($\frac{1}{4}$ per cent) are normally prescribed for insertion into the conjunctival sac, every hour if necessary. Where this does not suffice to suppress the aqueous exudate, prednisolone can be injected subconjunctivally, and given sytemically (as tablets, 5 mg. up to six times a day).

2. **Atropine,** which paralyses the ciliary muscle and iris sphincter, allows physiological rest and relief from the pain due to spasm; it also encourages the blood-flow, and dilates the pupil so that any posterior synechiae will be formed well away from the central (visual) area. One per cent atropine sulphate drops or ointment are normally given 2–3 times a day, reducing to $\frac{1}{2}$ per cent daily as the inflammation wanes. Atropine-sensitivity frequently develops, especially when the stronger concentrations are used, leading to eczema of the lids and conjunctiva (Fig. 35); in such cases many weaker substitutes are

available, particularly hyoscine; homatropine causes only a transient pupillary dilatation and a negligible ciliary paresis, so that it is rarely used except as a diagnostic aid in ophthalmoscopy and retinoscopy. These mydriatics, by forcibly dilating the pupil, may very exceptionally provoke an acute glaucoma in eyes that happen to have very shallow anterior chambers; so after a homatropine mydriasis for ophthalmoscopy it is wise to constrict the pupil again with a drop of eserine.

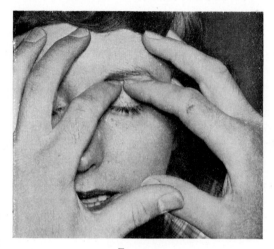

Fig. 41.
Digital Tonometry.

3. **Heat** will relieve the pain and allay the inflammation. It is most readily provided by seating the patient before a bowl of nearly-boiling water, and giving him a wooden spoon around the end of which is wrapped a bandage containing some cotton-wool; the patient dips the end in the water, and gradually approximates it to his closed eye, so keeping the eye as hot as he can bear, and when the pad becomes perceptibly cool it is dipped back in the water and the process is repeated.

4. **A Pad,** which keeps the lid firmly closed over the eye, will provide rest and relieve photophobia.

Any underlying disease should naturally have first attention, the patient should rest, and any complication of the iritis may require specific measures (e.g. a secondary glaucoma will need acetazolamide, and surgical drainage if uncontrolled).

ACUTE GLAUCOMA

Glaucoma signifies an increased intra-ocular pressure. The term was originally coined because of the grey-green colour as of a stormy sea that the waterlogged cornea transmits in an acute glaucoma, and it was later applied to the insidious 'chronic' form which was also characterized by a raised intra-ocular pressure but in which the front of the eye looked normal. Both acute and chronic glaucoma may be *secondary* to a manifest and specific eye disease which interferes with aqueous drainage (as iritis, or an intraocular tumour), but for the majority of cases no overt cause is apparent and these are labelled *primary*. Both acute and chronic glaucoma are rare before middle-age.

Primary acute glaucoma (or, more properly, 'closed-angle' glaucoma) is characterized by bouts of raised tension. These are largely precipitated by a protrusion of the iris root mechanically shutting off the recesses of the anterior chamber (from which the aqueous drains into the canal of Schlemm), since attacks are virtually confined to eyes with a very shallow anterior chamber, and consequently a very narrow drainage-angle; this protrusion may be due to an accumulation of aqueous behind the iris root, or to the natural thickening of the latter that accompanies pupillary dilatation, perhaps abetted by vasodilatation and oedema. Such congestive attacks are more common in the middle-aged, and occur especially in hypermetropes (the smaller eyeball having a proportionately shallower anterior chamber); the attacks themselves are often precipitated when emotion or fading light causes the pupil to dilate.

SIGNS AND SYMPTOMS

The congestive attack starts abruptly with severe pain in and radiating around the eye. The patient is prostrated, nauseated, and may even vomit, while vision may be reduced to a bare perception of light. On examination there is a dusky ciliary congestion, and the cornea appears steamy (due to the corneal oedema collecting under the epithelium as minute blisters). The congestion of the iris will make the anterior chamber more than usually shallow, and the iris itself will be seen (albeit darkly through the misty cornea) to be dull grey and patternless owing to the oedema; while the pupil is typically dilated, vertically oval, and fixed to light (Fig. 42, facing p. 44). The ocular tension is of a stony hardness.

When these bouts of ocular hypertension are mild and transient, they suffice only to cause a little oedema of the cornea without any pain or congestion, as a result of which the patient sees coloured haloes around lights—a *subacute glaucoma*. Such mild attacks do little, if any, damage to the retinal elements, but they are danger signals, since they may well be followed by the dramatic onslaught of the acute attack; while to the old-hand they may simply serve as benevolent reminders that the pilocarpine drops are overdue.

TREATMENT

Since the attack is precipitated by a swollen iris-root impeding drainage, the treatment seeks primarily to constrict the pupil and so disencumber the angle of the anterior chamber, and entails:

1. **Eserine** (1 per cent) or **Pilocarpine** (4 per cent) drops every 10–15 minutes for several hours.

2. **Acetazolamide** (Diamox), 250 mg. intramuscularly and thereafter t.d.s. by mouth. This drug inhibits aqueous production.

3. **Heat** (as 'Wooden-spoon' bathing, p. 48) relieves the pain and facilitates the absorption of the eserine.

4. **Pad,** Relieving the photophobia.

5. **Analgesics,** Even morphia may be merited for the pain.

Should these measures fail, a draught of **glycerol** (75 ml. in water or lemon juice) may well be effective in dehydrating the eye by its osmotic effect in the blood. The classical emergency operation of a 'Glaucoma Iridectomy' (in which a wide sector of the iris is excised), should rarely be required, as it is nearly always possible to soften and decongest such eyes by routine medical treatment, supplemented, if necessary, by intravenous mannitol, thus permitting a subsequent planned drainage operation, as for an unrelieved simple glaucoma (p. 66).

Once the attack has been controlled, or the subacute 'haloes' correctly diagnosed, a régime of pilocarpine drops (1–2 per cent b.d.) is necessary to maintain a constricted pupil, and so prevent a further congestive attack; but a Peripheral Iridectomy (making a small hole through the iris root, to allow free passage of aqueous between anterior and posterior chambers) may be a surer prophylactic, as well as avoiding the nuisance and slight darkening effect of the daily drops (which are generally needed in both eyes, since the tendency is normally bilateral).

Differential Diagnosis

	Acute Conjunctivitis	*Acute Iritis*	*Acute Glaucoma*
Pain	grittiness	moderate to severe	severe and radiating
Discharge	often purulent	slight reflex epiphora only	
Photophobia	mild	severe	moderate
Cornea	bright and clear	K.P.	epithelial oedema
Pupil	normal	constricted, fixed; later irregular from adhesions	dilated, oval, fixed
Iris	normal	muddy	greenish-grey
Tension	normal	normal (tender)	very hard (very tender)

ACUTE KERATITIS

Keratitis may be exogenous or endogenous. The former is much more common, since the cornea is exposed throughout life to a succession of minor traumata and the conjunctival sac is a favourite harbour for pathogenic bacteria; such an exogenous keratitis thus first involves the superficial corneal layers, and, since the epithelium has normally been disrupted, presents as a *corneal ulcer*. Endogenous keratites, due to systemic allergy or toxins, start deep in the cornea; they are an ill-assorted group deriving from a miscellany of discoverable and undiscoverable agents, but including one important clinical entity, due to congenital syphilis—*interstitial keratitis.*

CORNEAL ULCERS are generally of two main groups: (1) The small multiple *marginal ulcers* (Fig. 43), due to a severe conjunctival infection, usually with staphylococcus aureus, which transgresses the corneal margin; they are generally mild, clear away with routine antibiotic applications, and cause no ultimate impairment of vision. (2) The larger *central ulcer* (Fig. 44) which is usually single; this may be due to a pneumo-coccus that has been allowed to penetrate the corneal substance through an abrasion or alongside a corneal foreign body; more often nowadays it is a superficial but indolent 'dendritic ulcer'

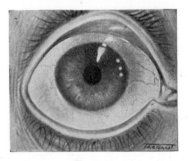

FIG. 43.

Marginal Corneal Ulcers. Catarrhal ulcers, secondary to a conjunctival infection. (Ainslie.)

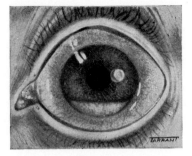

Fig. 44.

Pneumococcal Corneal Ulcer with a typical hypopyon, the ulcer is spreading medially beneath an overhanging edge.

(Fig. 45) provoked by the herpes simplex virus. Central ulcers also occasionally arise in degenerative conditions, as this area is farthest from the nutrient blood vessels at the corneo-scleral margins (e.g. in eyes devitalised by long-standing iritis, in keratites associated with skin diseases as acne rosacea, and in keratomalacia due to lack of vitamin A) and from over-exposure (e.g. where the lids cannot adequately protect the cornea, as in endocrine exophthalmos or facial palsy).

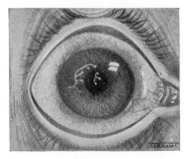

Fig. 45.

Dendritic Corneal Ulcer.

SIGNS AND SYMPTOMS

These are essentially a composite of the signs and symptoms of the underlying conjunctivitis (irritation, conjunctival injection, discharge), plus those of the mild iritis (boring pain, ciliary injection, impaired vision) promoted by the seepage of toxins through into the anterior chamber; the latter are more evident in the more infiltrating central ulcers, in which the exudation into the aqueous is so intense that it may gravitate as a hypopyon (Fig. 46). In addition the ulcer itself will be apparent as a cloudy opacity in the cornea; this can be confirmed to be an actual ulcer (and not just a scar from previous ulceration, in an eye which is injected for some incidental reason), by demonstrating that the overlying epithelium is deficient—since a drop of a vital stain such as fluorescein, followed by one of saline, placed into the conjunctival sac, will stain the exposed area bright green. When the ulcer is large and central, the visual loss will be correspondingly great.

Only the most severe corneal ulcers progress to perforation, such as those due to infantile gonococcal conjunctivitis

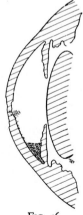

Fig. 46.

Section of Cornea with pneumococcal ulcer, showing hypopyon and purulent deposit on the posterior corneal surface.

(ophthalmia neonatorum) or the central ulcer caused by the rare but devastating contaminant of eyedrops—pseudomonas pyocyaneus. Even then the iris generally falls forward to plug the hole, and the inflammation may then subside, leaving an anterior synechia up to the base of the scar (Fig. 76).

TREATMENT

This correspondingly entails a combination of the treatment for the underlying conjunctival infection (**antibiotic** drops, etc.) plus that for the secondary iritis (**atropine, heat, pad,** but not corticosteroids, which delay epithelial regeneration). In the case of dendritic ulcers, the specific antiviral drops of idoxuridene are effective if given frequently (every hour) in the early stages; and steroid drops have an especial danger in promoting an extension of the ulcer.

Various further measures may be required if, as is all too frequent, the ulcer is indolent. **Carbolization** (painting the whole corneal surface with pure carbolic acid, after anaesthetic drops, and with care to avoid any excess reaching the conjunctiva) often expedites recovery. A **Tarsorrhaphy** (suturing the lids together) may be required to give added protection if the corneal sensation is lowered, as in the fairly common herpes zoster of the ophthalmic division of the trigeminal nerve ('neurotrophic keratitis'), or else where the lids are prevented from covering the eye as after a facial palsy ('neuroparalytic keratitis'), or when mechanically impeded from doing so as in a severe exophthalmos.

INTERSTITIAL KERATITIS is one of the ultimate stigmata of the congenital syphilitic (although milder forms very occasionally occur in acquired syphilis, tuberculosis, etc.); it develops about puberty, and one eye follows its fellow a few months later. Both corneas become very oedematous, and subsequently pink with the ingrowth of new blood vessels from the adjacent sclera (Fig. 47); after some months of pain and virtual blindness, the periphery of the cornea begins to clear, leaving only a diffuse cloudiness in the central area, so that

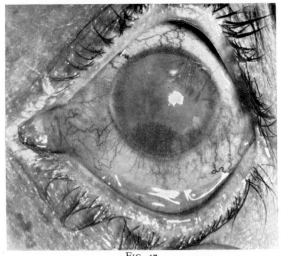

FIG. 47.

Interstitial Keratitis. Generalized haze with ingrowth of pallisade of deep
corneal blood-vessels. (Cook.)

the majority of cases regain enough vision to read ordinary
print. The actual cause is probably an anaphylactic reaction to
the spirochaetal endotoxin, and the treatment is thus palliative
until the disease has run its course, entailing drops of **corticosteroid** (which can reduce the intensity of the oedema and vascularization until the attack is finally over, and thereby reduce the
ultimate scarring) and **atropine** (an intense iritis is a normal, if
invisible, accompaniment). Antisyphilitic therapy is usually
given, but only in the hope that it may prevent a subsequent
gummatous or nervous lesion.

When the attack is over, the resulting corneal scars ('nebulae'
if faint, or 'leucomata' if dense) are especially amenable for
replacement by grafts from the cornea of a healthy cadaver eye.
This operation of corneal grafting or 'keratoplasty' (Fig. 48)
although rather uncertain in its results, may dramatically restore
the sight; cadaver eyes are in short supply, as the cornea becomes
unsuitable for grafting within a few days unless it is 'deep-

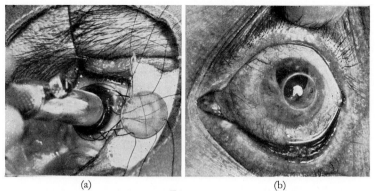

(a)   (b)
FIG. 48.
Keratoplasty. (a) Trephining the cornea, after insertion of sutures and splint.
(b) The graft in situ: an 'optical iridectomy' had previously been performed.
(Philps.)

frozen'; but eye-banks are now established in London and other major cities. In England patients may bequeath their eyes for grafting, and the eyes can then be taken without obtaining the consent of their executors, providing the surviving spouse or relatives do not object.

SCLERITIS, or 'episcleritis'—since the vascular superficial laminae of the sclera are principally involved, is one further cause of painful red eye. It arises generally as a form of collagen degeneration, essentially comparable to rheumatic nodules elsewhere in the body.

The eye develops an area of injection, at first sight resembling a conjunctivitis, but this is fairly localized to one part of sclera, which is indurated at that point (Fig. 49, facing p. 44), and the patient experiences a constant dull ache, rather than a 'grittiness' on movements of the upper lid; in the more severe cases there are signs of an underlying iritis. The disease lasts a few weeks, with a tendency to relapses; but the discomfort can be requited with topical steroids (also given systemically, if necessary) and these can be used symptomatically till the bout passes. Oral salicylates and topical heat are also helpful.

E

CHAPTER V

GRADUAL LOSS OF SIGHT IN QUIET EYES

BLINDNESS in England is caused, in the main, by three diseases:—
Cataract (23 per cent), Glaucoma (13 per cent) and Senile
degeneration of the macula (27 per cent); except for the less
common 'acute' glaucoma and the very occasional secondary or
juvenile forms of these three diseases, they all develop insidiously
in the elderly; but whereas cataract can be remedied, glaucoma
can only be arrested, and retinal degenerations ruthlessly progress. To these three major causes of a gradual loss of sight may
be added the various forms of optic neuritis, and intracranial
lesions which are outside the exclusive domain of ophthalmology.

CATARACT

The lens is avascular, and its cells (apart from the anterior epithelium) lose their nuclei and therefore cannot divide; their only
function is to remain transparent, and their only response to any
insult—developmental mishap, inflammation, disordered metabolism or radiation—is to become opaque, so forming a 'cataract'. However, the large majority of cataracts represent a simple
senile change, analogous to the degeneration of other epidermal
derivatives such as the whitening of the hair, and some degree
of lens opacity is found in the majority of patients over 60.

SIGNS AND SYMPTOMS

The cardinal symptom is a gradual failure of sight, and the
cardinal sign is a white opacity within the pupil (Fig. 50). In the
early stages the cataract may be barely visible on direct illumination, but presents ophthalmoscopically as a silhouette against the
red fundus reflex, often localized to the lens nucleus, or else as
flakes, dots or sector-shaped opacities within the lens periphery
(Fig. 51).

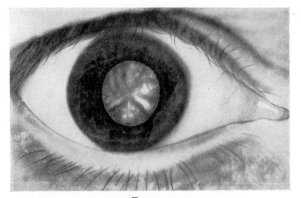

FIG. 50.

Mature Cataract: a white opacity within the pupil

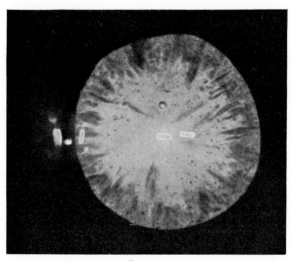

FIG. 51.

The wedge-shaped peripheral opacities of a cortical cataract, presenting an ophthalmoscopy as silhouettes against the red fundus reflex.

TREATMENT

Opacification of the lens is irreversible, since the protein becomes denatured as in a hard-boiled egg; so the only treatment of such an opacity is to remove it by operation. This can be performed at any age or any stage in its development, and is normally advised whenever the cataract becomes a sufficient impediment to the patient's normal activities—generally when it interferes with reading (this corresponds roughly to the time when the vision in the better eye is reduced to 6/18), and then the cataract is removed from the worse eye, if (as is usual) both are affected. Beneath the age of 35 it will suffice to tear open the lens capsule with a needle (cf. Fig. 54), so that the aqueous can mix freely with the opaque soft lens matter, which will gradually be washed away into the blood stream; such 'needlings' may

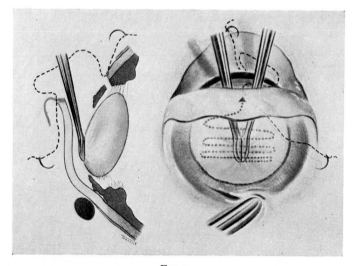

FIG. 52.

Cataract extraction. The Intracapsular technique, grasping the thin capsule with forceps, gradually dislocating it by side-to-side movements, and then somersaulting the entire lens out through the limbal incision. Counter-pressure is applied by a blunt hook at the lower corneal margin.

need to be repeated several times before all the opaque lens matter disperses. However, over the age of 35 the nucleus of the lens becomea increasingly sclerosed, and this solid nucleus must then be extracted through an incision in the eyeball along its corneo-scleral margin. The standard form of this operation involves the removal of the entire lens—an 'intra-capsular extraction'—grasping its tenuous capsule with forceps or, more simply and securely, by adhering the lens periphery to a freezing 'cryo-probe'; and then gently lifting the whole lens out of the eye (Fig. 52). The older method—an 'extra-capsular extraction'— is technically easier, the capsule being simply torn open (as in the operation of 'needling') and the hard lens nucleus squeezed out through the incision (Fig. 53). This extra-capsular method has the disadvantage that the capsule which has been left behind

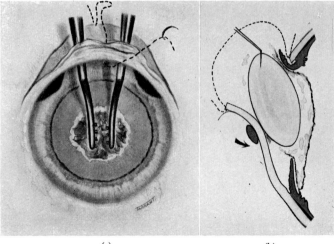

(a)   (b)

FIG. 53.

Cataract extraction. Extracapsular technique (a) preliminary avulsion of central part of the anterior lens capsule. (b) expression of the lens nucleus through this gap in the capsule and out through the limbal incision, easing it away with a sharp hook as it emerges.

will need to be punctured several weeks later (a 'capsulotomy' Fig. 54), before the light rays can have unimpeded access to the retina. After cataract extraction, thick convex spectacle-lenses are needed to replace the convex 'crystalline lens' that has been removed from within the eye, and then full vision can usually be restored.

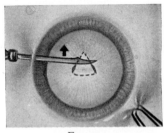

FIG. 54.

Capsulotomy. Division of the thickened posterior capsule or 'after-cataract' with a needle-knife; here a tongue-shaped flap is being cut, which will fall downwards with gravity and leave a clear central gap in the capsular remnant.

CONGENITAL CATARACTS vary in size from an entirely opaque lens to the occasional dots that can be seen in most normal lenses and cause no visual impediment. Sometimes they are specifically attributable to maternal disease, thus cataract is an almost invariable sequel to rubella when this is contracted within the first eight weeks of pregnancy, and a 'lamellar cataract' (shaped like a plate in the posterior lens cortex, with its thickened rim generally just concealed by the pupil margin—Fig. 55) is often the result of a lowered blood calcium just before or after birth.

Binocular congenital cataracts should be removed (by 'needling') within a few months of birth, if they are dense enough to render the infant almost blind and so prevent the development of macular fixation; otherwise, or if uniocular, a needling is generally merited about the age of six.

SECONDARY CATARACTS may result from **trauma** (concussion, or an actual rupture of the lens capsule from a perforating wound), **intra-ocular inflammation** (by impeding its metabolism, or by frank toxins from a protracted irido-cyclitis), **endocrine upset** (adolescent diabetics may be blinded by a sudden snowflake-like deposit throughout the lens cortex, although this has become rare since the widespread use of insulin, and must be distinguished from the ordinary senile cataract to which diabetics are especially prone; or cataracts may form in aparathyroidea, due to lowered blood calcium), **radiation** (X-rays and infra-red rays).

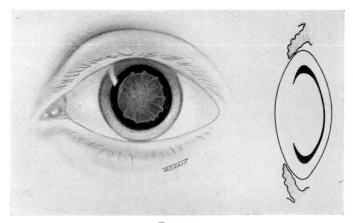

FIG. 55.

Lamellar Cataract. The position of this plate-shaped opacity within the lens is shown in the diagram alongside.

SIMPLE GLAUCOMA

When the intra-ocular pressure is raised very gradually over many months, all the acute manifestations of a congestive glaucomatous attack are lacking, since the eye remains white and painless, but the damage to the retinal elements, which in the acute attack is dramatic, is here so insidious that it is easily overlooked by the patient (or by the untrained practitioner) until much of the sight is irretrievably lost.

The aetiology of simple glaucoma is obscure, since the anterior chamber is of normal depth and there is no overt obstruction to the drainage angle. It is probably, in the main, a senile sclerotic process of the smaller intra-ocular vessels, and secondarily of the ocular tissues; in the anterior segment of the eye this sclerosis obstructs the aqueous outflow, and so elevates the intra-ocular pressure, while posteriorly it leads to an ischaemic atrophy of the fibres in the optic nerve-head which causes both the atrophic cupping of the disc and restriction of the visual fields. The elevated pressure thus damages the sight only indirectly, by aggravating the ischaemic changes of the posterior segment.

SIGNS AND SYMPTOMS

1. *The intra-ocular pressure is raised,* although the eyeball is not so hard as in an attack of acute glaucoma.

2. *The vision is gradually destroyed.* This loss starts as a blind patch—a 'scotoma', which soon forms an upward or downward

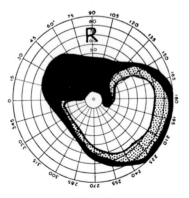

FIG. 56.

The field-loss in simple (chronic) glaucoma: Encroachment of the upper nasal sector has become confluent with the 'arcuate' scotoma which extends upwards from the normal blind-spot. (The blacked-out area represents that part of the normal visual field which has been totally lost, and within this is a stippled area where vision is present but impaired.)

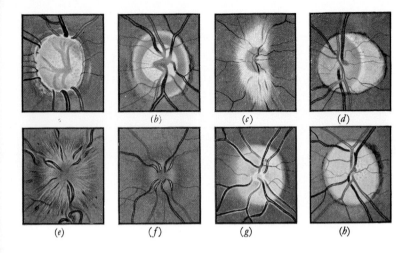

FIG. 57 (*see pages* 6, 65, 72, 92).

(*a*) Glaucomatous cupping of the optic disc.

(*b*) Physiological cupping of the optic disc.

(*c*) Opaque nerve fibres spreading onto the adjacent retina.

(*d*) The optic disc in myopia—enlarged by a crescent of exposed sclera.

(*e*) Papilloedema.

(*f*) The optic disc in high hypermetropia ('pseudo-papilloedema').

(*g*) Post-neuritic ('secondary') optic atrophy.

(*h*) Simple ('primary') optic atrophy.

extension of the normal blind-spot, and reaches to join an indentation of the peripheral field in the upper or lower nasal quadrants (Fig. 56); and it progresses till only a small circle of the central vision remains, although within this surviving island the acuity is barely affected. Finally, the eye becomes quite blind.

3. *The optic disc is cupped*, and at the same time becomes white and 'atrophic' (Fig. 57a). This must be differentiated from physiological cupping, which is simply an exaggeration of the central pit, does not reach the disc margin, and is not atrophic (Fig. 57b).

TREATMENT, as for the acute bouts of congestive glaucoma, consists essentially in attempting to control the tension with miotic drops (pilocarpine 1–4 per cent or eserine $\frac{1}{4}$–$\frac{1}{2}$ per cent, daily up to t.d.s.), and where this fails—as evidenced by a persistently raised pressure or a continued encroachment of the visual fields on charting every few months—a surgical decompression of the eye. Diamox is less valuable here than in acute

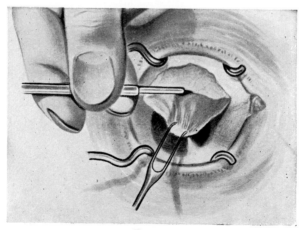

FIG. 58.

The trephine operation. After reflecting a conjunctival flap, the disc of corneo-sclera is excised by rotating the trephine between the fingers.

glaucoma, but should supplement the miotics in cases with a high tension which are less suitable for surgery. The standard operation is the sclerectomy, in which a small piece of sclera at the upper corneal margin is removed (as well as a knuckle of the underlying iris root), so that the aqueous under pressure can filter out through the hole and disperse into the subconjunctival lymphatics; traditionally this piece of sclera is excised by a circular 'trephine' (Fig. 56), but nowadays a knife and scissors are usually preferred. As an alternative, a wick of iris tissue may be partially freed and drawn out through the corneo-scleral incision, to produce there a spongy filtering scar—an 'iridencleisis'. Sometimes these drainage operations need repetition, or need to be supplemented by further miotic drops; and even then the degenerative process may continue, albeit retarded, to destroy the sight.

CONGENITAL GLAUCOMA arises from maldevelopment at the drainage-angle of the anterior chamber. The soft infantile sclera distends under the increased intra-ocular pressure, so that these swollen eyes look ox-like and the condition is thus called *Buphthalmos* (Fig. 59). A similar line of treatment is required,

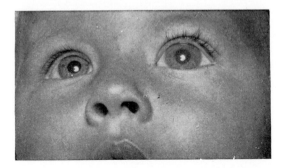

FIG. 59.

Buphthalmos. The left eyeball is distended, and its cornea rendered hazy with oedema. (Lister.)

although the visual results are poor in the more established cases.

DEGENERATION OF THE RETINA AND CHOROID

A miscellany of degenerative fundus changes, beyond the range of treatment, are a common cause of gradual visual loss in old age: they are ascribed to a genetic lowering of vitality of the neural or vascular elements of the choroido-retina, and generally labelled 'dystrophies' or 'abiotrophies'. They are usually localized to the macular area.

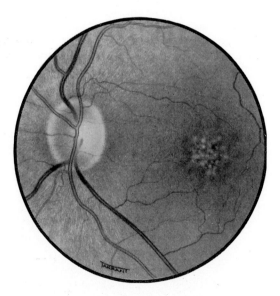

FIG. 60.

Senile Macular Degeneration.

Senile macular degeneration presents clinically with an insidious bilateral *central scotoma*; and the corresponding area of macula becomes mottled with pigment (Fig. 60), a change that is easily overlooked in the earliest stages, but in some cases the whole area may become swollen with exudate or spattered with haemorrhage and haemorrhagic residues. Such patients may be assisted by certain optical devices (as telescopic spectacles), but the involuting mind adapts tardily, and a simple hand-magnifying-lens often serves them best. These macular degenerations may occur in young adults or even infancy, having then a more obvious hereditary-familial basis, being proportionately more rapid, and, in the youngest groups such as Tay-Sachs disease, being accompanied by degenerative changes in other tissues that are usually fatal. Similar pigmentary degenerative changes at the macula may be the legacy of prolonged dosage with toxic drugs, such as chloroquine.

Retinitis Pigmentosa is the commonest of the dystrophies that cause a loss of the *peripheral* vision; it sometimes presents

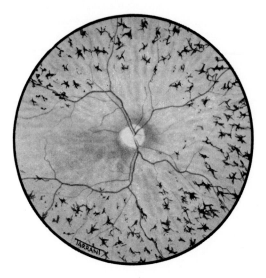

FIG. 61.

Retinitis Pigmentosa. The 'bone-corpuscle' pigment-deposits are restricted to the retinal periphery.

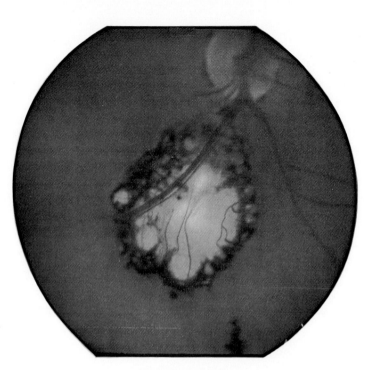

FIG. 62 (*see page* 69).
Scarring from foci of choroiditis. (Hansell, *Brit. J. Ophthal.*, *37*.)

with a night-blindness, since the retinal periphery is largely responsible for night-vision. The fundus shows a striking scattering of black pigment, in patterns resembling bone-corpuscles, at first involving the equatorial region but finally over all but the posterior pole (Fig. 61). Degeneration of the retinal elements starts in adolescence, progresses remorsely, and is attested by an increasing retinal pigmentation and a deepening pallor of the optic disc as the ganglion cells die.

Atrophy of the choroido-retina is also a classical result of foci of **choroiditis**; and the exposed white sclera, together with occasional areas where the retinal pigment-epithelium has proliferated, may give an appearance resembling the foregoing primary retinal degenerations, except that the areas involved are usually irregular and, if bilateral, rarely symmetrical (Fig. 62); the visual loss is also stationary and dates from a bout (often unrecognized) of impaired vision due to the vitreous exudation during the acute attack. The aetiology of acute choroiditis is essentially the same as that of iritis (generally unknown, but serological tests attribute a fair proportion to toxoplasmosis); and the treatment is similar except that, since there is no pain or photophobia, heat and pad are unnecessary, and even atropine has probably little influence on its evolution; topical corticosteroids barely penetrate to the posterior segment of the eye, so prednisolone (5–10 mg. t.d.s.) is usually prescribed until the acute attack subsides.

A similar choroido-retinal atrophy occurs in **high myopia** (or 'progressive myopia'), when it is restricted to the area of the macula and around the optic disc. There is proportionate loss of central vision, which is often sudden if small retinal tears or haemorrhages appear.

Both acute choroiditis and high myopia are characterized by opacities in the vitreous, caused respectively by inflammatory exudate and degenerative changes in the gel as the eyeball elongates, and when these opacities are sufficiently dense, or so placed that they cast discrete shadows on the retina, they become visible to the patient, and float with each movement of the eye. Minor 'floaters' occur in healthy eyes as wisps and dots, which are barely visible except against an even light background; they have no pathological significance, and are known as *muscae volitantes* (flitting flies).

DAMAGE TO THE OPTIC PATHWAYS

OPTIC NEURITIS

Inflammatory or degenerative foci may arise in the optic nerve from a variety of causes. Very occasionally they are placed so near its anterior end that the engorgement may be visible ophthalmoscopically on the optic disc as a *papillitis* (this closely resembles a papilloedema due to raised intra-cranial pressure, but the latter is accompanied by a negligible loss of sight), otherwise it is a *retro-bulbar neuritis*, and the only visible change arises later as a pallor of the optic disc—an 'optic atrophy' which may be very indefinite if only a few of the axon bundles have been destroyed.

Acute Optic Neuritis is generally due to the inflammatory foci of Disseminated Sclerosis or related (? virus) neuropathies. The axon bundles from the central regions of the retina are

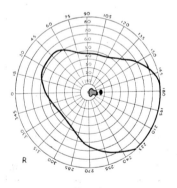

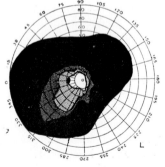

FIG. 63.

FIG. 64.

Field loss in optic neuritis. Paracentral scotoma, as in tobacco amblyopia.

Field loss in optic neuritis. Peripheral loss, as in Tabes.

usually damaged, so that the blurred vision can be shown (by mapping the visual fields) to be due to a central or paracentral scotoma (Fig. 63). In the early days the eyeball may be tender or eye-movements painful due to the stretching of an inflamed optic nerve. The inflammation recedes after a week or two, leaving little, if any, visual damage, but further bouts are liable, and ultimately a pallid disc may develop as the sight is whittled away.

Chronic Optic Neuritis is generally due to poisons, and thus known as 'toxic amblyopia', although this includes endogenous toxins as in tabes and avitaminosis A and B. In the majority of forms the optic nerve-fibres from the central area are similarly affected, again producing a central or paracentral scotoma, and they are often accompanied by signs of a peripheral neuritis elsewhere in the body; the minority (including organic arsenic and tabes) depress vision generally, so that the impulses from the less sensitive retinal periphery become submerged, and the visual fields show a peripheral constriction (Fig. 64). These poisons include tobacco, methyl and ethyl alcohol, quinine, lead and arsenic; although presenting as an optic atrophy from axon degeneration, the damage is probably inflicted on the parent cells of these axons—the ganglion cells of the retina. The visual loss is usually insidious, as in the commonest form—the tobacco amblyopia which follows prolonged and heavy use of cheap pipe tobacco, but may indeed be acute if large amounts of the poison are ingested as with methyl alcohol and quinine. Abstinence is the essential treatment, combined with adequate doses of vitamin B12.

PRESSURE ON THE OPTIC NERVE may arise from injury (as skull fractures), haemorrhage, aneurysm (typically an intracavernous aneurysm of the internal carotid artery, with coincident oculomotor palsies), tumour (typically a pituitary tumour, causing bitemporal hemianopia, or less commonly, a tumour of the optic nerve itself). And the principal feature will be an encroachment on the visual field corresponding to the distribution of fibres within the optic nerve, at the chiasma, and in the optic tracts (p. 6). Ophthalmoscopically, the optic disc may show evidence of such lesions either as an oedema and engorgement (papilloedema) due to a raised pressure within the optic nerve sheath, or as an optic atrophy following destruction of the optic nerve fibres.

Papilloedema (Fig. 57e) is characterized by an oedema that elevates the disc forward from the retina, tends to fill in the central (physiological) optic pit, and blurs the disc margins, and by a venous engorgement that makes the disc redder than normal and often spattered with small haemorrhages. It is generally due to pressure on the central retinal vein within the optic nerve sheath from a raised intracranial pressure (as from a cerebral tumour); occasionally the disc oedema is simply part of a generalized retinal oedema (as in malignant hypertension—Fig. 66) or of a focal inflammation (a papillitis).

Optic Atrophy—an atrophy of the optic nerve fibres—is revealed by a pallor of the disc due to an atrophy of their supporting capillaries. This may be a *simple optic atrophy* (Fig. 57h, facing p. 65), when the damage is due to local pressure, toxins, ischaemia, or inflammation (retro-bulbar neuritis or meningitis); or else it may follow a papilloedema, when it is styled a *post-neuritic optic atrophy* (Fig. 57g, facing p. 65), and the disc margins and central pit then seem less well-defined, with glial tissue also sheathing the emergent vessels. A third group is the *consecutive optic atrophy* caused by damage to the parent ganglion cells of the retina (as in choroido-retinitis, dystrophies or central artery occlusion).

CHAPTER VI

SUDDEN LOSS OF SIGHT IN QUIET EYES

THE gradual extinction of sight in one eye may well be over-looked by the incurious or obtuse patient, and the presence of a blind eye is then suddenly discovered when the seeing eye happens to be occluded; but a sudden loss of sight rarely passes unnoticed, however painless. This is normally the result of a vascular mishap—either blockage of the end-arteries or 'end-veins' of the retina, or a copious intra-ocular haemorrhage; or else only a part of the visual field may be lost, following a retinal detachment or a vascular mishap involving the optic tracts or radiations—including the relatively common homonymous hemianopia that follows a thrombosis of the posterior cerebral vessels. Since the former group devolve in the main from retinal arteriosclerosis and the related retinopathies, these may first be briefly considered, although to some extent they fall more within the ambit of general medicine.

RETINAL ARTERIOSCLEROSIS

The following pathological changes in the retinal arteries can be discerned (Fig. 65):

1. **Spasm**—often intermittent and localized; the blood columns then appear narrowed (the vessel walls themselves are normally invisible), and the retina may appear opalescent from oedema (the retina itself is also normally invisible, and the fundus background is formed by the blood in choroidal vessels with their associated pigment, faintly screened by the single layer of the retinal pigment-epithelium).

2. **Sclerosis**—a thickening of the arterial walls which gives the heart an added load, although if a raised systolic pressure can be maintained, retinal function is unimpaired. This is shown ophthalmoscopically by the vessel walls themselves becoming opaque, with at first a bright surface reflex ('copper-wire arteries'), which may later even conceal the underlying blood-

column ('silver-wire arteries'); at the same time the hardened arteries press on the veins at their crossings, interrupting, and later deflecting the venous column.

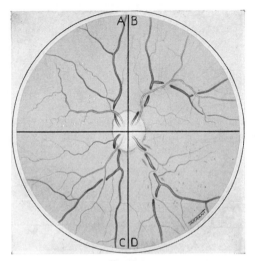

FIG. 65.

Retinal Arteriosclerosis. The four quadrants illustrate the sequence of vascular changes, with increasing evidence of pressure at the arterio-venous crossings, increasing attenuation and irregularity of the arteries, and finally scattered haemorrhages and exudates in the retina.

3. **Constriction** of the blood column, when intimal proliferation encroaches on the lumen.

4. **Retinopathy**—with *haemorrhages,* which being superficial are flame-shaped (since they spread tangentially among the fibres of the inner layer of the retina, as these converge towards the optic disc), and also some small *hard exudates.* These various deposits may cause little visual impairment and constantly clear away to be replaced by haemorrhages and exudates elsewhere.

MALIGNANT HYPERTENSION differs essentially from the foregoing fundus picture of benign hypertension in showing

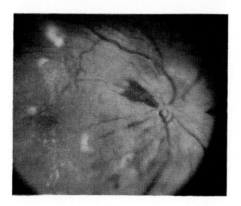

FIG. 66 (*see page* 75).

Retinopathy in Malignant Hypertension. Fundus photograph showing gross oedema of optic disc and adjacent retina, with superficial haemorrhages and scattered 'cotton-wool exudates'.

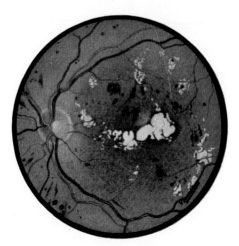

FIG. 68 (*see page* 76).

Diabetic Retinopathy, with small deep haemorrhages and 'hard exudates'.
(Whittington.)

a generalized arterial spasm, leading to gross retinal oedema which may spread onto the disc (as papilloedema), along with areas of retinal necrosis ('cotton-wool patches') (Fig. 66).

RENAL RETINOPATHY may augment a hypertensive-arteriosclerotic retinopathy when the toxic metabolites due to reduced kidney function further damage the retinal arterial walls, rendering them more permeable; so that oedema, then exudates, and finally haemorrhages appear. These latter are all variable in amount and constantly changing; the exudates characteristically form a fan-shaped pattern around the macula, and may entirely disappear before death (which is usually less than six months distant when the retinopathy develops) (Fig. 67).

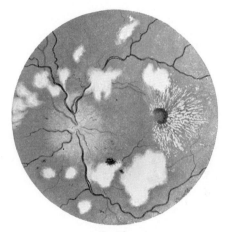

Fig. 67

Renal Retinopathy, with haemorrhages, 'cotton wool exudates' and linear 'hard exudates' radiating like a fan around the macula.

DIABETIC RETINOPATHY develops 10–20 years after the onset of the diabetes; the majority of cases are thus middle-aged, so that the signs of diabetic retinopathy are again generally complicated by the coincident signs of retinal arteriosclerosis. The primary lesion is a multitude of 'micro-aneurysms'; these are minute varicosities, just visible ophthalmoscopically, which later tend to leak and form haemorrhages, small and dark because they are deep within the retinal substance—producing the characteristic 'dot and blot' appearance (Fig. 68, facing p. 75). The exudates, which appear some years later, are also small, with 'hard' irregular edges, like pieces of cheese. These changes become gradually more profuse as the sight is destroyed, and blindness is often precipitated by a massive haemorrhage into the vitreous; however, the retinopathy of diabetes, unlike the other forms, has no worse prognosis for life.

OCCLUSION OF THE CENTRAL RETINAL ARTERY

The central retinal artery may be blocked by spasm, by degenerative changes within its wall, or very rarely by an embolus; arterial occlusion is thus most common in the elderly

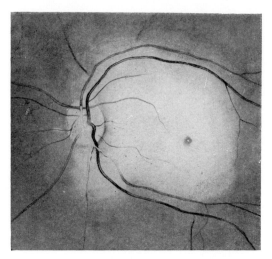

Fig. 69.
Occlusion of the central retinal artery.

arteriosclerotic, but may occur in the young adult with cardio-vascular disease.

Sudden blindness is here associated with a classical fundus picture (Fig. 69), the arteries becoming transformed into narrow threads, and the whole fundus appearing milky white as the oedematous retina loses its transparency; a day or two later a 'cherry-red spot' appears at the macula (where the retina is thin and the red choroid shows through, in contrast to the adjacent pallor), and by the time the retinal oedema has faded an optic atrophy is generally apparent.

When occlusion of the artery or its branches is simply due to spasm, this may relax within an hour or two and vision return, otherwise blindness is complete, although an aberrant vascular supply to a patch of retina may occasionally salvage an island of sight. Antispasmotics are usually administered, but with little prospect of success if the block has persisted more than a few hours.

Occlusion of the central retinal artery (or, less often, of the vein) is a common sequel in the elderly to Giant-cell arteritis. This diagnosis should always be suspected, and will often be confirmed by finding a raised E.S.R. Treatment with systemic steroids may then prevent a similar catastrophe in the fellow-eye.

OCCLUSION OF THE CENTRAL RETINAL VEIN

The central retinal vein is generally occluded by pressure of its escort artery at the optic disc, especially in the presence of venous congestion; occasionally occlusion is due to a toxic endophlebitis. Thus it is similarly more common in the elderly arteriosclerotic, but again may arise in younger adults (usually women).

Sudden blindness again develops, but a little less abrupt and less complete; and there is an equally arresting fundus picture, with haemorrhages scattered riotously over the whole retina, irregular and superficial like bundles of straw alongside the retinal veins, which are themselves tortuous and very engorged.

After a few weeks the haemorrhages gradually clear, and little trace of the initial onslaught ultimately remains, apart from the occasional but pathognomonic formation of new anastomotic vessels on the disc; however, the sight, which initially permits little more than 'counting fingers', may show scant improvement. Treatment is of no avail.

The tranquil course of resolution is interrupted after about three months in nearly 20 per cent of cases by an acute secondary glaucoma, which expunges the little sight that remains; the pathogenesis of this is obscure and treatment also of little profit except for the symptomatic relief of pain.

As often as not venous occlusion (with a secondary thrombosis) is limited to one of the four principal trunks (Fig. 70), with the

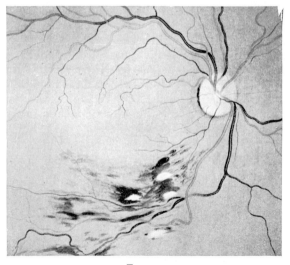

Fig. 70.

Occlusion of the lower temporal branch of the central retinal vein.

obstruction visibly beginning at an arterio-venous crossing, and the damage will then be confined to the appropriate sector, the macula being involved if either the upper temporal or lower temporal veins are affected; but here the recovery of sight is generally greater, and there is no risk of a subsequent glaucoma.

VITREOUS HAEMORRHAGE

Retinal haemorrhages are seen to be a major component of the various retinopathies; they similarly develop in many blood diseases wherein haemorrhages are especially liable (anaemia, purpura, etc.), and particularly in an idiopathic disease of young adult males attributed to tuberculous periphlebitis and named 'Eales' Disease'. When severe, they irrupt into the vitreous cavity (a particular feature of Eales' disease, in which vitreous haemorrhages occur every few months over a period of several years); but sometimes they are restrained behind the hyaloid membrane that bounds the vitreous, and then appear as a characteristic **pre-retinal** or **subhyaloid** haemorrhage—forming an even film, with an outline which is circular but may develop a flattened upper margin as the blood corpuscles gravitate

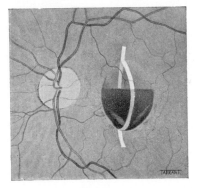

FIG. 71.

Pre-retinal ('sub-hyaloid') haemorrhage, with its upper fluid level, contained between the posterior surface of the vitreous and the inner surface of the retina (these two surfaces are here illuminated by the vertical beam of light which is coming in obliquely from the right-hand side).

downwards (Fig. 71). The dispersal of vitreous haemorrhages is slow, but may be completed after many months; only when they are very extensive or often repeated do they become organized, leaving the eye partially or completely blind.

RETINAL DETACHMENT

In embryology the retina is formed by the invagination of an optic vesicle, the outer layer persisting as the single-celled layer of 'pigment epithelium', and the inner layer proliferating to form the rods, cones and the various cell-relays. The cavity of the optic vesicle persists as a potential space between these layers; and, if the inner layer should rupture, vitreous can pour in through the hole and open up this space, by displacing the visual layer of the retina forwards, as a 'retinal detachment'. Such ruptures generally occur from trauma, or else in the elongating eyes of high myopia where the retina may fail to stretch as much as the sclera.

SIGNS AND SYMPTOMS

The rods and cones over the detached area are thus separated from their choroidal blood supply and will ultimately die, so that to the patient it seems as if a curtain was descending (or ascending, if the detachment started above—corresponding to the lower visual field), and central vision is abruptly lost when the detachment spreads across the macular area.

Ophthalmoscopically the detached retina becomes apparent as an opalescent sheet 'ballooning' well forwards into the vitreous, and the initiating tear is usually visible, with the brilliant red choroid shining through it (Fig. 72).

TREATMENT

If untended, the detachment normally becomes complete, and the eye blind. In about three-quarters of the cases the detachment can be arrested by sealing the retina back to choroid all

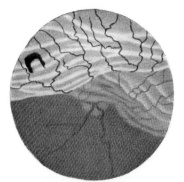

Fig. 72 (*see page* 80).
Retinal Detachment.

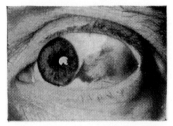

Fig. 75 (*see page* 84).
Subconjunctival Haemorrhage.

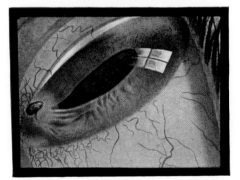

Fig. 76 (*see page* 87).
Perforating Corneal Wound near the lower corneal margin, this has become
plugged by 'prolapsed' iris, which forms a black knuckle externally.
Hamblin.)

around the hole, so blocking any further seepage of vitreous fluid between the layers. This is achieved by invaginating the sclera and choroid towards the detached retina in the region of the retinal hole, and then the choroid and retina are made to adhere by the coagulating effect of a diathermy or freezing terminal placed at appropriate sites on the overlying sclera. Such an adherence can also be attained by an intense light-beam directed through the pupil ('photocoagulation'), and this simple procedure alone may suffice if the retina and choroid are already virtually in contact. Even in successful cases, a re-detachment is liable, usually initiated by some mild trauma to the head or a physical effort such as stooping, especially in the myopic cases where the retina is already thin and degenerate; bed-rest is thus advised after the operation (and also pre-operatively to prevent any interim extension of the detached area).

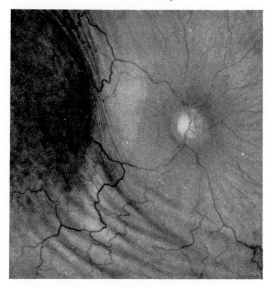

FIG. 73.

Malignant melanoma, as seen on ophthalmoscopy, with the dark choroidal mass above, and a secondary fluid detachment below.

SECONDARY RETINAL DETACHMENTS are occasionally caused by a massive exudate between the two layers (as in the toxaemia of pregnancy) or a rapidly progressive neoplasm of the retina or choroid.

The two common primary malignant tumours of the eye are the **malignant melanoma** of the choroid, and a **retinoblastoma** of the retina. Both progress quickly till they fill the eyeball, often presenting when they obstruct the drainage angle and induce glaucoma; a third stage is that of local extra-ocular spread, and a fourth of distant metastases—the melanoma generally reaching the liver, and the retinoblastoma travelling up the optic nerve into the brain. The clinical picture of these tumours is otherwise very contrasting; the melanoma is uniocular, generally presenting in the middle-aged, as a dark oval mass, often concealed beneath

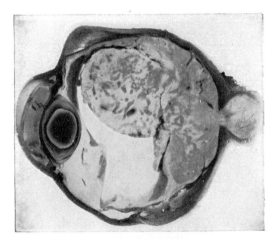

FIG. 74.

Retinoblastoma. Section of an eye excised for advanced retinoblastoma; this is seen to be half-filling the vitreous cavity, and extending up the optic nerve which is strikingly swollen; the lens has become cataractous and dislocated, while neoplastic cells largely fill the anterior chamber. (From the museum at the Institute of Ophthalmology.)

a secondary retinal detachment (differentiation from a primary detachment is thus imperative but often difficult) (Fig. 73); while the retinoblastoma (Fig. 74) presents in early infancy as a white mass behind the pupil (a similar appearance may be the result of intra-uterine endophthalmitis, or of retrolental fibroplasia—a retinal maldevelopment largely due to administration of excessive oxygen to premature babies). Eyes containing either of these tumours must be enucleated forthwith;[1] retinoblastomata are, however, often bilateral (and also familial), in which case an attempt should be made to save the second eye by destroying its tumour with X-radiation or (if small enough) by coagulation.

[1] An eye may need to be removed in order to save life, sight or pain; in other words—(1) for malignant tumours; (2) if sympathetic ophthalmitis threatens; (3) if it is blind and painful; in the last group an attempt is usually made simply to relieve the pain by a retrobulbar injection of alcohol, unless the globe is purulent, ruptured or disfiguring.

CHAPTER VII

THE INJURED EYE

ALTHOUGH the overhanging orbital ridges afford great protection against direct injury from any large object, small particles notoriously find their way into the eye, with effects which are disproportionately irritating in the case of corneal foreign bodies, or damaging in the case of perforating wounds.

CONTUSION OF THE EYE

The following lesions may be caused:

Haematoma of eyelids, the classical 'black eye': blood oozes freely into the loose subcutaneous tissues, and then lingers there for about two weeks. Apart from an inspection of the eyeball to exclude further damage, no treatment is necessary.

Subconjunctival haemorrhage (Fig. 75, facing p. 80). This usually involves only one sector and does not appear to extend backwards into the orbital tissues (if there is no such limitation posteriorly, it may be a forward extension from an intra-orbital haemorrhage, and so may signify a fracture of the skull that involves the orbital walls). The large majority of these haemorrhages are spontaneous, especially in arteriosclerotics, or less commonly are due to a sudden venous congestion as in whooping cough. They are symptomless, and, again, take about two weeks to disperse.

Corneal abrasion. The epithelium is readily stripped off the corneal surface, often over a large area, leaving a very painful, irritable eye. The abrasion may be difficult to see, unless an irregularity is noticed of the corneal light-reflections (as from the window), but it can easily be demonstrated by instilling a drop of vital stain such as fluorescein followed by a drop of normal saline, which renders the denuded area bright green.

The epithelium quickly regenerates, provided the eyelids are kept closed by a pad and bandage (to splint the cornea, and at the same time relieve pain and photophobia), and the abrasion remains uninfected (a drop of antibiotic solution should be used to prevent the abrasion turning into a corneal ulcer). Such healed abrasions occasionally re-open spontaneously many months later ('recurrent abrasions').

The iris. Contusions frequently cause a little *bleeding* into the anterior chamber—a 'hyphaema', blood gravitating to the lower segment, and dispersing a few days later; only if the whole anterior chamber is filled with blood is there a danger that the aqueous drainage may be obstructed, and the resultant secondary glaucoma will then require surgical relief (incision at the corneal margin so that the blood can be evacuated). Major *tears* may occur at the iris root (an 'iridodialysis', the pupil then becoming D-shaped) or at the sphincter; and even without a visible tear, the sphincter may be paralysed for weeks or longer as a 'traumatic mydriasis'. These tears show little attempt at healing, but rarely interfere with sight. Atropine drops are sometimes prescribed until the eye is quiet.

The lens. A *concussion cataract* may form, similar to that induced by heat or radiation, and merit removal. *Dislocations* are usually partial, so that the lens is drawn to one side with consequent visual distortion; occasionally the suspensory ligament is completely broken and the lens falls backwards into the vitreous (leaving a tremulous, unsupported iris—an 'iridodonesis'), or slips through the pupil into the anterior chamber (inducing a painful spasm of the pupil behind it, and a secondary glaucoma by obstructing the aqueous drainage). Partial dislocations of the lens are sometimes found as a bilateral congenital mishap, often in association with arachnodactyly and other systemic defects.

The Retina. Contusions of the eyeball may cause a transient retinal *anaesthesia* (a 'black-out'), without objective changes. More severe blows may cause retinal oedema which is ophthalmoscopically visible as a whitish cloud obscuring the red fundus pattern; this normally clears in a few days, but may leave a little residue of pigment-proliferation with an equivalent scotoma of depressed vision, which typically is found at the macula, as in the retinal burns of an 'eclipse-blindness'.

Retinal *haemorrhages* generally remain small, and cause visual embarrassment only if overlying the macula; occasionally they irrupt into the vitreous where the loss of vision may be almost complete, and with the ophthalmoscope the red fundus reflex is correspondingly almost or completely obscured. The latter take many months to clear, and if extensive or repeated, the clot may organize and permanently impair the sight. *Tears* usually occur at the anterior limit of the retina, and may lead to a retinal detachment which spreads across the macular area some weeks later. Sometimes only the choroid is ruptured, causing a white streak (of exposed sclera) in the fundus, usually near the disc or macula.

The **optic nerve** may be torn or compressed in fractures involving the orbital walls, and blindness is usually immediate, complete and permanent, the dense pallor of a primary optic atrophy becoming ophthalmoscopically visible several weeks later.

PERFORATING INJURIES

Wounds of the **eyelids** require prompt suturing, with exact restoration of the torn lid margin; the blood supply of the lids is so profuse that such lacerations heal well and hardly ever become infected. If the lower lacrimal canaliculus is torn, special measures are needed to prevent a permanent barrier to the drainage of tears. Conjunctival lacerations require suturing with fine silk only if they are very extensive, as they heal rapidly.

Burns of the eyelids are more serious because of the risk of subsequent distortion of the lids with cicatrization (entropion or ectropion) and hence of corneal ulceration through exposure. The treatment entails inspection of the eyeball to exclude further damage and to remove any foreign bodies, with instillation of atropine and antibiotic ointment, before the reactionary oedema renders the lids difficult to separate. The skin should be dusted with sulphonamide-penicillin powder, and further routine measures may be needed if the burns are extensive. In the case of chemical burns, the eye should be copiously irrigated, as by immersing the head promptly in a bucket of water; while with alkali burns the risk of a subsequent symblepharon is great, and further attention will be as needed.

Perforating wounds of **Cornea** or **Sclera** are often small and barely visible, but they should be suspected if the history is suggestive and any intra-ocular lesion is apparent. Perforating wounds require surgical closure if they are gaping, and since the iris will generally have fallen forwards to plug any corneal wound through which the aqueous has escaped (Fig. 76, facing p. 80), this 'prolapsed' iris must first be excised, before the wound is closed. As immediate treatment, atropine and antibiotic drops should be instilled.

The presence of a retained foreign body must first be excluded— a special liability after use of a hammer and chisel. Sometimes such foreign bodies are visible; otherwise they can be demonstrated radiographically, or signalled by a sharp pain when they are shifted in the field of a giant magnet. Small particles that have sufficient force to penetrate the tough wall of the eyeball are generally metallic and then usually magnetic, so that they can be extracted with the giant magnet, otherwise their evacuation is often difficult and hazardous.

Retained iron particles will gradually dissolve, but the brown pigment is then dispersed through the intra-ocular tissues ('siderosis bulbi'), and the sight is gradually destroyed. Other metals tend to provoke suppuration; while some foreign bodies, like glass, may remain inert for years.

Perforating injuries to the **lens** will disrupt the lens capsule and cause a cataract.

Pyogenic Infection of the eyeball often follows such injuries, and pus can be seen to accumulate in the anterior chamber as a hypopyon. The inflammation generally recedes, leaving a shrunken, blind eye—'phthisis bulbi'; but the pus may spread into the scleral lamellae, and the globe finally rupture. These cases need antibiotic therapy, systemically and by subconjunctival injection; but when a panophthalmitis is established, little hope remains of saving the eye, and the pain and toxaemia lend an urgency to its removal. This is normally performed by an 'evisceration' in which the disorganized contents are scooped away from the scleral envelope (the latter being left behind to prevent the risk of disseminating infection into the orbital contents, and up through the sheath of the optic nerve). In other circumstances the eye is removed by an 'enucleation' (Fig. 77) in which the conjunctiva is divided by a circular

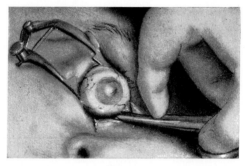

Fig. 77.

Enucleation of the eye. The rectus muscles have been severed, and the optic nerve is being divided with scissors, after dislocating the eyeball forwards between the blades of the speculum. (May and Worth's *Diseases of the Eye*.)

sweep over the rectus insertions, which are then themselves cut, allowing the eyeball to be prolapsed, and the optic nerve to be reached and divided. Sympathetic ophthalmitis has been noted as an occasional devastating sequel to perforating wounds, especially when they involve the ciliary region and are not purulent, and the eye may need to be removed if the inflammation shows little improvement after three weeks, as a prophylactic against involvement of its fellow eye. Otherwise the eye is excised only if grossly disorganized, or blind and persistently painful.

Non-perforating foreign bodies generally become impacted on the cornea where they provoke a characteristic irritation, augmented by every movement of the eyelid. They should be removed (after anaesthetizing the cornea with a drop of amethocaine); a piece of cotton-wool will occasionally suffice for this if they are very superficial, but usually they need to be excavated with a flattened needle (a blunt 'Spud', that simply hammers the projecting end of the embedded particle, is still frequently preferred from timidity, ignorance or habit). Thereafter, a drop of antibiotic should be instilled, with a further drop of atropine (1 per cent) if the crater is deep and the eye very irritable; and the lid should be kept closed with an eye-pad until the epithelium has healed. If no foreign body can be seen on the cornea, the upper lid should be everted (Fig. 4) as such particles are frequently caught in a horizontal groove beneath the tarsus, where they abrade the cornea with each blink, and whence they can easily be whisked away with the ball of the finger.

CHAPTER VIII

REFRACTIVE ERRORS

THE normal eye is so shaped that rays of light from a distant object are made to converge on passing the convex corneal and lens surfaces, and are brought to an exact focus on the retina. Nearer objects can then be brought into focus by a contraction of the ciliary muscle allowing the lens to become more spherical.

There are four types of 'refractive error' in which the images are not focused correctly on the retina: the inadequacy of accommodation that comes in middle-age (Presbyopia), variations in the length of the eyeball (Hypermetropia and Myopia), and variations in the corneal curvatures between different meridians (Astigmatism). And these may all be remedied by appropriately-curved spectacle lenses. A pinhole aperture will also neutralise the blurring caused by a refractive error; and this provides a useful test to indicate whether a poor visual acuity is simply due to such an optical distortion rather than an organic impediment to sight.

Presbyopia—The range of focusing (or 'accommodation') decreases throughout life as the lens becomes stiffer with age, so that the nearest point that can be brought into focus on the retina recedes beyond the normal reading-range at about the age of 45, and presbyopia is then said to have set in. This can be compensated by weak convex spectacles, which will require strengthening every few years.

Hypermetropia—For the *Short* eyeball, distant objects can be brought to a focus on the retina, which here lies in front of the normal focal point, by using a convex spectacle lens (Fig. 78). In the youthful hypermetrope such a focusing is normally done spontaneously by accommodating the lens of the eye, but this leaves less reserve of fattening for near-vision, so that fatigue-symptoms on near-work may develop (usually in adolescence), or a decreasing near-range of vision may be encountered before

DISTANCE   NEAR

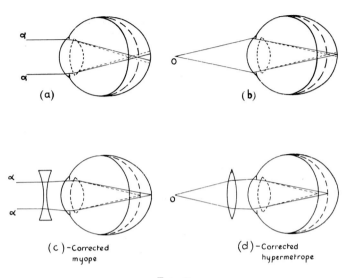

(a)   (b)

(c) –Corrected   (d) –Corrected
myope   hypermetrope

FIG. 78.

Refraction in the hypermetropic and myopic eye. The outlines represent the short (hypermetropic) and the long (myopic) eyeballs, with the intermediate (interrupted) outline of the normal-lengthed, normal-sighted eye. The effect of accommodation in bringing forward the point of focus is shown by the dotted line.

The posterior principal focus, which falls onto the retina in the normal-lengthed eyeball both in distance-vision (a) and near-vision + accommodation (b), only falls onto the hypermetropic retina with accommodation alone (a), and onto the myopic retina with near-vision in the absence of accommodation (b).

(c) shows the myope, with his concave spectacle lens pushing his focal point backwards towards his backward-placed retina, so as to allow clear distance-vision.

(d) shows the hypermetrope, with his convex spectacle lens bringing his focal point forwards towards his forward-placed retina , so as to allow clear near-vision.

the usual age of 45. These merit the assistance of convex spectacle lenses for close work (Fig. 78d).

Myopia—For the *Long* eyeball, distant objects can only be brought to a focus on a retina, which here lies behind the normal focal point, by a concave spectacle lens (Fig. 78c). However, near objects can still be focused on the retina by inhibiting the normal reflex of accommodation (Fig. 78b), myopes are thus 'short-sighted'. In more severe cases of myopia the eyeball may continue to elongate throughout life ('progressive myopia') leading to a retinal degeneration (Fig. 69), or even detachment; but the majority cease to progress after adolescence, and a little reduction of the myopia may even follow in late middle-age.

It may here be noted that myopic eyeballs often do, in fact, look large, even exophthalmic; and through the ophthalmoscope the optic disc in myopia seems proportionately large and pale—simulating an optic atrophy (Fig. 57d), whereas the optic disc in hypermetropia looks small and pink—often simulating a papilloedema ('pseudo-papilloedema'), (Fig. 57f).

Astigmatism—Here the eyeball is flattened, generally from above downwards, but sometimes sideways, or along an oblique axis. Vision is then proportionately blurred both for near and distance, irrespective of accommodation, and visual fatigue (ocular headaches) may occasionally accrue. In the rare cases where the astigmatism is sufficient to cause symptoms, these are compensated by spectacle lenses with an appropriately different curvature in the two meridians.

TESTING OF REFRACTION is performed either subjectively (finding by trial-and-error which lens gives best visual acuity, and ordering the strongest convex lens or weakest concave lens that permits full vision) or objectively (determining by 'retinoscopy' what strength of lens is required to neutralize the movement of a beam of light reflected from the fundus); this latter technique requires considerable practice, but is more secure than the subjective method, and is the only way of refracting the woolly-minded adult or inarticulate child. Such a retinoscopy can only be accurate if the ciliary muscle is at rest; so a mydriatic should first be instilled, and for the powerful ciliary muscles of children repeated applications of atropine are usually needed.

SPECTACLES are thus required either to improve visual acuity, or else to relieve an 'eye-strain' or headaches (but only when such symptoms may be legitimately attributed to the particular refractive error that is present), and such spectacles should be used thereafter only if they materially improve the vision or specifically relieve these fatigue-symptoms. It must be emphasized that the vast majority of headaches bear no relationship to refractive errors, and also that the eyes themselves can never be damaged by uncorrected or wrongly-corrected refractive errors[1]. Refractive errors are due to anatomical variations, and the progress of myopia is likewise genetically determined, so that refractive errors cannot be remedied or their progress curbed by medicaments, diet, exercises, or any other fanciful nostra.

Spectacle lenses are thus convex (for presbyopia or hypermetropia) or concave (for myopia); and since the curve of the cornea is rarely exactly the same in all meridians, this associated astigmatism (generally too slight to demand treatment of itself) is then also corrected by giving the spectacle lens an added convexity or concavity in the appropriate meridian. The strength or 'power' of such lenses is measured in terms of dioptres (1 'D' $= 1$/focal length of the lens in metres). Finally, a prism can be incorporated into such lenses to compensate a slight malalignment of the eyes ('latent squint'), but this is, in fact, hardly ever indicated. Spectacle lenses can be darkened, like sun-glasses, and very occasionally a genuine photophobia justifies this, but the vast majority of dark glasses are sought in the hope of protecting a frail psyche or concealing a guiltful one from the harsh or revealing light of day.

Contact lenses are spectacle lenses that slip beneath the eyelids and thus are barely visible externally. These are optically

[1] The only occasion where glasses may help to prevent impairment of sight is in some rare cases of amblyopia in small children, where the suppression of function is central rather than ocular. In all other cases spectacles are justified only when they sufficiently improve the vision or comfort to outweigh their nuisance-value.

necessary for the very rare cases of corneal irregularity, optically useful for high myopia, and uniocular aphekia, and cosmetically convenient for the low myopes who count their glasses a social blemish. Nowadays the large majority of lenses provided are the small 'corneals', fitted readily (albeit often expensively) from stock, and well tolerated for 8–10 hours.

TROPICAL OPHTHALMOLOGY

THE foregoing chapters aim to cover the field of ophthalmology as encountered in the Western world; but students in tropical and subtropical countries will need to supplement these by a basic knowledge of the eye-diseases peculiar to their own regions, and which may there provide the principal causes of loss of sight.

The eyes of such tropical and subtropical peoples have certain differences in their normal responses that should be noted. They usually become presbyopic much earlier—generally around the age of 35. Their iris, loaded with pigment cells, dilates less readily and less completely with mydriatics—a barrier to easy fundus examination and retinoscopy; and the exuberant pigment cells may spread, particularly along the penetrating scleral vessels, to give the spurious appearance of conjunctival melanosis or melanomata. This same exuberance probably explains the tendency for operative fistulae in simple glaucoma to become blocked and require repetition. On the other hand, the eyes of most coloured races are generally more resilient, and withstand a raised intra-ocular pressure with less damage to the fields of vision; and they heal more readily after injury or operation than their less pigmented fellows.

Hypovitaminosis is so widespread in the undernourished countries that it may justly be included as a 'tropical disease', and deficiency of vitamins A and B is the commonest cause of blindness in many such areas.

Vitamin A is a fat-soluble alcohol deriving from the vegetable pigment carotene. A deficiency causes dessication and keratinization of skin and mucosae, which in infants particularly involves the eye, leading to rapid and permanent blindness through corneal perforation. At first the conjunctiva becomes dull, leathery and rather wrinkled, while the corneal epithelium follows suit ('xerophthalmia'), and ulceration follows. The inflammatory response is slight, so the eye may not attract attention until the iris is seen to be bulging through a wide gap in the lower central cornea. If sloughing of the cornea is threatened, a large intramuscular dose (100,000 i.u.) of vitamin A may avert this disaster and save the eye; later on the vitamin can be given orally (50,000 units a day), together with dietary control (especially adequate milk).

In adults, where the skin changes are more marked than those of the cornea and conjunctiva, the other ocular manifestation—night blindness—is often the presenting feature. This can be crudely tested by noting a relative delay in discerning objects, such as the ability to count fingers, when the room is suddenly darkened.

The *vitamin B* complex is a group of water-soluble enzymes needed for intracellular metabolism; they are found in most animals and plants, and especially in cereals and yeasts. A lack of thiamine (B_1) provokes a polyneuritis, paraesthesia, weakness and loss of reflexes, including any form of ocular palsy. These signs may be submerged, in the 'wet' form of beriberi, by a presenting oedema due to heart failure.

Lack of riboflavine (B_2) presents (some weeks after any associated signs of B_1 deficiency) with angular stomatitis, glossitis, scrotal dermatitis, vascularizing keratitis, and, later, a retrobulbar neuritis; the latter may leave a permanent central or paracentral scotoma, with some corresponding optic atrophy.

Epidemic Dropsy is another nutritional disease, which provokes a characteristic glaucoma. It is due to poisoning by argemone oil (from seeds of the Mexican poppy), which is commonly used in India and Pakistan in cooking and for anointing the body. This poison produces a gross generalized dilatation of capillaries, including those of the uvea; a glaucoma develops in consequence, with a high tension and persistent haloes, but with little conjunctival congestion and only a very gradual field loss. The glaucoma may persist, even after the poison is excluded, and it will then require control with oral acetazolamide (miotics are ineffective), or an operation if there has been a significant field loss.

Viral Keratoconjunctivitis. *Trachoma* (p. 38), although very rarely seen in England except among immigrants, is almost world-wide in distribution, and in the Middle East few children escape some pathognomic scarring of the lid and cornea. Vaccines are still experimental, but the cicatricial entropion that is the usual cause of blindness can be rectified by a variety of quite simple plastic operations that evert the inturned upper lid-margin with its ingrowing lashes.

Epidemic keratoconjunctivitis occurs only sporadically in England, but as widespread outbreaks in tropical countries. It presents with an oedematous conjunctiva (developing follicles on its tarsal surface), and tiny spots on the cornea ('superficial punctate keratitis'). It is caused by adenovirus type 8, which, unlike the virus of trachoma, is outside the range of sulpha and antibiotic drugs; atropine and a pad normally allow resolution in about two weeks, otherwise the corneal infiltrate may spread and damage the sight, especially if topical steroids are used.

Leprosy is found in most humid countries of the tropics and subtropics, and is usually contracted during childhood (adults having a high resistance). The eyes are involved in about a quarter of both clinical types.

The *tuberculoid (neural)* form shows scattered patches over the skin which are pale, dry and variably anaesthetic; the lids are commonly affected, with loss of lashes and eyebrows, and the skin may become so stiff and contracted that the lids cannot close, especially if the facial nerve is also damaged. Progressive corneal ulceration from exposure is thus an almost certain sequel unless the eye is protected by a tarsorrhaphy.

In the *lepromatous* form, patches also appear on the lids, but these are less well-demarcated and only an inch or two in diameter. They become increasingly prominent, forming nodules that produce ptosis rather than a lid retraction, while loss of the eyelashes and eyebrows is again a feature. In this type of leprosy the bacilli may invade the eye itself, causing episcleral nodules or a deep corneal infiltrate; many cases indeed show very fine punctate corneal deposits which are symptom-free (and which lack any of the vascularization that characterizes trachoma and ariboflavinosis). The infection may spread to provoke iritis or choroiditis, or even a frank leproma may develop within the anterior chamber.

Onchocerciasis, due to the filaria Onchocerca volvulus, is a frequent cause of blindness in Central Africa and Central America. The microfilariae (transmitted by the Jinja fly) spread beneath the skin and frequently (in about a third of cases) invade the cornea, causing infiltrates that resemble snowflakes; in severe infections these opacities may coalesce and obstruct the sight, or a secondary iritis may develop; while the sight may also be damaged by choroido-retinal degeneration and optic atrophy (less certainly due to onchocercal infection). These ocular changes improve markedly after treatment with diethylcarbamazine (Hetrazan).

Many other tropical diseases can occasionally damage the sight, but in most cases this is too rare or coincidental to deserve emphasis here. Thus the skin of the lids commonly partakes in any generalized urticaria (as with *schistosomiasis*), and commonly suffers the bites of *insects* and *spiders*; *ticks* may adhere so firmly to the eyelid that only a hot probe or a dab of chloroform will dislodge them, just as an adherent *leech* will need a touch of salt before it releases its hold. Such bites and stings can similarly involve the conjunctiva, which may also find itself a receptacle for fly larvae (*myiasis*), or be invaded by the caterpillar hairs that provoke an *ophthalmia nodosa* (these may even penetrate the cornea to provoke nodules on the iris!). The cornea may likewise be damaged by *ant* bites (mainly in infants) or by the projected venom from 'spitting' *snakes*. Corneal ulcers also feature in *cholera*, where exposure ulceration often develops during periods of semi-coma, or in *malaria* where dendritic ulceration is a common sequel. To all these may be added a retinue of fundal changes (the retinopathy of *sickle-cell anaemia*, and so on); but, as was said in our opening paragraph, although ophthalmology is a small speciality, the whole field of medicine lies within its frontiers.

OPHTHALMIC QUESTIONS FROM SOME RECENT 'FINAL' EXAMINATION* PAPERS IN SURGERY

Cambridge, M.B., B.Chir.

Give the causes, signs, symptoms and treatment of detachment of the retina.

A wicket-keeper is struck in the eye by a fast-rising ball. What immediate injuries may result, and how would you investigate them in hospital?

Discuss the value of the ophthalmoscope in surgical diagnosis.

Discuss . . . (a) The differential diagnosis of iridocyclitis.

Describe very briefly how you would deal with the following cases attending your surgery in private practice.
. . . (a) Abrasions of the cornea.

Describe briefly how you would deal with the following conditions occurring in a country practice.
. . . (a) Foreign body in the conjunctival sac.

Write short notes on . . . Acute glaucoma [twice].

,,   ,,   ,,   ,,   . . . Lacrimal duct obstruction.

,,   ,,   ,,   ,,   . . . Iridocyclitis.

,,   ,,   ,,   ,,   . . . Squint in childhood.

,,   ,,   ,,   ,,   . . . The differential diagnosis between acute conjunctivitis and acute iritis [iridocyclitis].

* Acknowledgements are due to the authorities of the Universities of Cambridge, Oxford and London, and to the Committee of Management of the Examining Board in England for permission to reproduce these questions.

Oxford, B.M., B.Ch.

Discuss the diagnosis and treatment of acute glaucoma.

What is glaucoma? How is it treated?

Write short notes on ... Exophthalmos.

London, M.B., B.S.

Give the symptoms, signs and treatment of acute glaucoma.

Describe the causation and treatment of conjunctivitis.

Conjoint Examining Board in England for R.C.P. and R.C.S.

State how you would deal with a patient alleged to have a foreign body in the eye.

Discuss the aetiology, diagnosis and treatment of corneal ulcer.

Discuss ... (a) The differential diagnosis of iridocyclitis.

Describe the management and complications of injuries to the eye.

Describe the orbit and its contents, excluding the internal anatomy of the eyeball.

Describe the causes, diagnosis and treatment of conjunctivitis.

Write short notes on ... Cataract [twice].

,,   ,,   ,,   ,,   ... Keratitis.

,,   ,,   ,,   ,,   ... Acute Glaucoma.

,,   ,,   ,,   ,,   ... Acute Iridocyclitis.

,,   ,,   ,,   ,,   ... Corneal Ulcer [twice].

,,   ,,   ,,   ,,   ... Optic Atrophy.

,,   ,,   ,,   ,,   ... Ectropion.

,,   ,,   ,,   ,,   ... Proptosis.

,,   ,,   ,,   ,,   ... Glaucoma [twice].

,,   ,,   ,,   ,,   ... Ectropion

,,   ,,   ,,   ,,   ... Conjunctivitis.

INDEX